STRETCHING
to Stay Young

Simple Workouts to Keep You Flexible, Energized, and Pain-Free

JESSICA MATTHEWS

Illustrations by Christian Papazoglakis

ALTHEA
PRESS

To my amazing husband and my incredible mother.
Thank you both for your unconditional love and support
that keeps me grounded and flexible in my approach to life.

STRETCHING TO STAY YOUNG

CONTENTS

PART THREE: THE WORKOUTS

Introduction

For more than 16 years, I've been in the business of helping people move better, feel better, and enjoy life to its fullest. I became interested in health and fitness after I witnessed firsthand the devastating effects of chronic diseases, such as diabetes, on the health of my family. I wanted to help myself and my loved ones have a better quality of life, so I set out to learn how healthy lifestyles—including regular physical activity—can improve our well-being. It quickly became clear to me that a career in fitness was my calling. So, at a young age, I made the decision to focus my academic pursuits and professional work on educating and inspiring others to live healthier, more active lives.

As a physical education major, group fitness instructor, and personal trainer, I spent most of the early part of my career deepening my understanding of the physical body. I taught an assortment of group cardio classes, including step aerobics and cardio kickboxing, and developed customized resistance-training programs for clients. Meanwhile I was studying technical topics, such as exercise physiology and biomechanics, as part of my undergraduate work.

Although I had learned about flexibility training from books and understood how stretching worked, it wasn't until I attended my first yoga class that I truly realized just how important flexibility is to overall health and wellness. At the time I did mostly cardio and strength-based workouts, as many people do, leaving little to no time for stretching. As I continued to neglect stretching before and after my workouts, I noticed that the high-impact exercise classes I was teaching, not to mention the long hours I spent studying, taking classes, and writing papers, were taking a toll on me and causing a constant feeling of tightness.

I will never forget that first time I stepped foot on my yoga mat and how humbled I was by my extreme lack of flexibility. Let's just say I was far from being able to touch my toes! Once I was stretching regularly, however, I began to move more easily—not just while exercising but in my everyday life as well. I increased my range of motion and gained immense flexibility, reducing the aches and pains I had become accustomed to. In addition, the personal time I spent stretching and breathing each day taught me the beauty of slowing down and tuning in, while also giving me the chance to mentally navigate the busyness and unforeseen events in my life with greater ease.

With this book, I hope you find what it took me so long to find for myself: a way to improve your fitness, health, and well-being. The wisdom I share with you here is rooted in the most up-to-date research and science. I have tried to set the record straight on many of the common myths that exist about stretching and provide an assortment of easy-to-follow stretches and flexibility-training routines to empower you to live the life you deserve.

PART ONE

The
SCIENCE

Everyone Stretches

Like many animals, we humans are meant to *move*. In fact, our bodies are uniquely designed to perform a wide range of movements. Yet, because of advances in transportation and technology, we move less throughout the day than in the past. We take elevators instead of climbing stairs. We drive to the local store and hope to get the closest parking spot possible instead of just walking. We ride lawn mowers instead of pushing them, and use snowblowers instead of shoveling snow. And we exchange countless e-mails with colleagues instead of walking over to talk to them face-to-face. All this leaves us sitting for hours at a time.

For each stretch included in this book, I've included easy-to-follow, numbered steps describing how to properly perform the movement, along with information about the benefits of each stretch and the key areas of the body the stretch targets. Make the most out of your stretching routine by using my tips on how to fine-tune your form and recommendations on how to vary the stretches using props or other forms of support (such as a table, wall, or chair) to meet your current fitness level, whether that means you want the stretch to be less intense or to produce more sensation.

Stretching is not a new concept. It's long been depicted throughout history in literature and artwork from around the globe. It has played a big part in physical activities—from centuries ago to more recent athletic and physical therapy programs and even combat training. When done correctly, stretching feels good, both physically and mentally, and improves your overall fitness. Regardless of your age, lifestyle, physical condition, or current level of flexibility, you can tailor stretches to meet your personal needs and goals. When you perform the stretches in this book regularly and with a sense of ease and relaxation, you will dramatically improve how you move and positively enhance your overall quality of life.

CHAPTER ONE

WHY STRETCHING WORKS

Flexibility is essential to physical fitness. We increase flexibility by stretching. By definition, *flexibility* is the range of motion around a joint. Each of our joints possesses its own degree of motion, so there is no true standard by which to measure "good" overall flexibility, such as the ability to touch your toes. Instead, as a healthy adult, you should be able to move each specific joint or series of joints fluidly, without stress or discomfort, through the full range of motion. Although your level of flexibility may be influenced by factors such as age (see chapter 3), the mechanics of flexibility are the same for all of us, as our muscles share the same structures and functions.

Know Your Muscles

We each possess three different types of muscle tissue in our body. In particular, skeletal muscle is the type that enables movement at the joints. Different muscles in the body produce different types of movements by shortening, or contracting, while other muscles must lengthen, or stretch. These opposing actions, ultimately, create your body's controlled movements.

In our workouts we often isolate muscles and movements. But our body is more of a kinetic chain, in which our individual muscle groups connect and work together as a single unit. For us to achieve fluidity and flexibility, this sense of balance among the various muscles must exist. When the muscles on each side of a joint share an equal degree of pull, we are able to move the joint freely in all directions. However, when one of our muscles becomes chronically tight and tense, weakening opposing muscles, we create wear and tear on various joints.

If your muscles are always tense, tight, and contracted, they weaken, causing you to become less limber. Poor posture, improper form when performing everyday tasks, repetitive movements, and spending long periods of time seated commonly lead to tight and tense muscles. This is why regular stretching using a variety of techniques is so vital to our overall health and well-being.

Studies Have Shown

Numerous studies show that we experience a better quality of life and other long-term benefits when we include various types of stretching in our daily routines. These benefits include the following:

DECREASED STIFFNESS According to a 2009 study published in the *Journal of Sports Sciences,* completing two 30-second bouts of static stretching may significantly decrease stiffness in your lower leg muscles.

IMPROVED FUNCTION Patients with knee osteoarthritis improved their range of motion and overall stability when they combined resistance-training exercises with static stretching and proprioceptive neuromuscular facilitation (PNF) stretching (see page 23), based on a 2009 study in the *Kaohsiung Journal of Medical Sciences.*

REDUCED PAIN Following a four-week stretching routine, women with non-specific neck pain reduced their pain levels, according to a 2007 study in the *Journal of Rehabilitation Medicine.*

ENHANCED PERFORMANCE A 2008 research study in the *Journal of Strength and Conditioning Research* found that a four-week, dynamic stretching warm-up program increased the agility, power, muscular strength, and endurance of athletes.

IMPROVED RANGE OF MOTION Individuals aged 60 to 70 may see significant improvements in their hip and shoulder ranges of motion when performing static stretching twice a week over the course of 13 weeks, according to a 2012 study in the *Journal of Strength and Conditioning Research.*

IMPROVED BALANCE Performing three 15-second bouts of static stretching targeting the major muscles of the lower body can produce significant improvements in your balance, according to a 2009 study in the *Journal of Strength and Conditioning Research.*

DECREASED ANXIETY AND DEPRESSION Following a seven-day comprehensive yoga program that included yoga-based stretches and mindful breathing techniques, participants with chronic lower-back pain reduced their anxiety, depression, and pain, according to a 2012 study in *Complementary Therapies in Medicine.*

The Benefits of Stretching

When you increase your flexibility, the benefits that follow will collectively enrich your life. With your improved range of motion, you will minimize aches and pains, improve your posture, and make physical activity more enjoyable. When your range of motion is restricted by tight, stiff muscles, this not only negatively affects how you move when exercising and when going about your everyday activities, but it also affects how you feel physically and mentally. Whether you are training with a specific fitness goal in mind or simply want to move with greater ease while working around the house, you will benefit in numerous ways from regular stretching.

STRESS REDUCTION AND PHYSICAL RELAXATION

If you experience chronic stress, your body goes through a number of undesirable responses, including feelings of anxiety, fatigue, and tension. Excessive muscular tension can increase your blood pressure, heart rate, and breathing rate and can also lead to pain and stiffness in your neck and lower back. In fact, 80 percent of us suffer from bouts of lower-back pain. But if we regularly perform stretching exercises, studies have shown we can reduce our stress, blood pressure, heart rate, breathing rate, and chronic neck or lower-back pain.

IMPROVED PHYSICAL PERFORMANCE

Regardless of your current state of physical fitness, stretching can benefit you in the short and long term. You may even experience short-term benefits immediately following your exercises and also after as few as 7 to 10 sessions in an intensive program, or as quickly as three to four weeks of stretching at least twice per week.

When you stretch, you can begin to show improvement in your muscle strength, agility, power, and speed. And when you include flexibility training as part of your well-rounded fitness routine—one that also includes resistance exercises to strengthen the muscles that affect your posture—your balance will improve, and, over time, your body will be in better alignment and your movements will be more pronounced and efficient.

PREVENTING INJURIES, MUSCLE SORENESS, AND CRAMPS

Although we don't have definitive evidence, some promising findings suggest that by stretching we may be able to prevent muscle soreness, relieve muscle cramps, and reduce our risk for injury. You can best prevent the aches and pains of sore muscles by gradually increasing the length and intensity of your exercise routines over a period of time, which is especially important when you're just starting out. Also, with a proper warm-up, you may avoid an intense soreness known as delayed-onset muscle soreness (DOMS), which typically shows up within one to two days of exercising. A proper warm-up increases your core body temperature and prepares your body for the movements to come and prevents strains, sprains, or rupturing cold muscles and tendons. And when you stretch regularly, your muscle cramps may become less frequent and severe, minimizing some of the discomfort we often experience in the body.

CHAPTER TWO

PROPER STRETCHING

When you stretch, you are working to increase your range of motion around your major joints and lengthen your muscles. A well-rounded flexibility-training routine includes stretches for the major muscle-tendon units of the ankles, legs, hips, back, torso, chest, shoulders, and neck, using a variety of stretching techniques and strategies.

What Makes a Good Stretch?

Quality movement involves nerves, connective tissue, and muscles all working together, so it's important to approach your stretching routine from a variety of angles. When you perform a "good" stretch, you basically move the two ends of a muscle—known as the origin and insertion—away from each other in the direction and arrangement of the muscle's fibers. For a muscle fiber to be lengthened, an external force must act on it. You can use anything from gravity, momentum, your body weight, resistive force applied by a partner, or a prop like a towel or a strap.

In addition to stretching muscles, we need to focus on fascia. *Fascia* is the densely woven, specialized web of connective tissue that provides structure and support to the body. It covers and unites all of the body's individual parts as one integrated unit. If your fascia is functioning as it should, your movements should feel unrestricted and pain-free. However, if you've been injured, have poor posture, or suffer repetitive stress within your body, your fascia will become tight and restricted, thereby limiting your range of motion.

STATIC STRETCHING

Often referred to as the most widely used form of flexibility training, static stretching is a passive approach to stretching. It involves stretching a muscle to the point where you feel mild discomfort, and holding that stretch at that point for an extended period of time, without moving. For static stretching, it is recommended that you hold the stretch for 15 to 30 seconds per repetition. If you are 65 years or older, or age 50 to 64 and experience chronic conditions or physical limitations that affect your physical fitness and range of motion, holding static stretches for a little longer, 30 to 60 seconds per repetition, may offer you greater benefits. In general, you should complete a total of 60 seconds of a flexibility exercise per joint, which can be done by repeating each flexibility exercise two to four times, depending on the length of time for each repetition.

DYNAMIC STRETCHING

Dynamic stretching is a more active approach to stretching that involves moving your joints through ranges of motion by using combined movements performed at controlled speeds. Commonly part of warm-up routines in fitness and sports, this type of stretching is basically your "rehearsal" opportunity in which your nervous system and muscles—known as the neuromuscular system—work together to prepare for the more intense exercises or activities to follow. You should begin with basic range-of-motion movements, both forward and backward (such as rolling your shoulders) before you add side-to-side and rotational movements. Ideally each dynamic stretch you perform should be done at a steady pace for a total of 10 repetitions.

PNF

Proprioceptive neuromuscular facilitation, known as PNF, is a specialized stretching technique that developed from physical rehabilitation methods. This approach combines tension in the muscle produced with little to no movement at the joint, known as isometric muscle contractions, along with static stretches. While you may come across different variations of PNF stretching, one common approach is the contract-relax method, which involves contracting the muscle you are targeting and then relaxing and stretching it with the assistance of a partner or equipment such as a towel or strap.

To perform PNF stretching, you contract your muscle for 3 to 6 seconds and follow it up with 10 to 30 seconds of static stretching per repetition. By following the contraction with a static stretch, you activate the muscle on one side of your joint, which allows the opposing muscle to become restricted, effectively stretching it.

SELF-MYOFASCIAL RELEASE

Although not technically a stretching technique, self-myofascial release will improve your joint range of motion. It releases tightness within your fascia, improving flexibility in the underlying muscle(s) you're targeting. While trained health and fitness professionals can apply certain techniques, known as myofascial release, you can perform these techniques on your own using a tool such as a foam roller. A foam roller looks like a pool noodle and comes in different levels of firmness for various levels of intensity and sensation.

You can apply pressure to tender areas of the body by performing small, continuous back-and-forth movements on a foam roller for 30 to 60 seconds. If an area of your body is especially tender and it is painful to perform the back-and-forth movements, you can place the foam roller directly over, or close to, the affected area, depending on your pain tolerance, and simply hold it there to apply pressure.

How to Stretch

The American College of Sports Medicine (ACSM) recommends performing flexibility-based exercises at least two or three days per week, with daily stretching being the most effective. You should hold passive static stretches to the point of mild tension or slight discomfort to enhance your joint's range of motion, but *never to the point where you feel pain.*

Interestingly, our muscles have built-in safeguards that protect them. When you stretch a muscle too quickly or intensely, your body reacts with an involuntary response known as the stretch reflex, in which your muscle contracts to protect itself from injury. While this built-in safeguard is helpful, you should still use measured movements and proper form to ease into and perform stretches safely and correctly so you avoid causing pain or injury and to get the most out of each stretch.

WARMING UP

Properly preparing yourself for physical activity—both physically and mentally—is just as important, if not more so, than performing the activity itself. With the right approach, you can create a well-rounded warm-up routine that prepares your muscles for the sport or activity to follow. This helps reduce your risk of injuries by addressing any underlying muscle imbalances you may have and enhancing your range of motion. Although there is no one "right" way to warm up, there are some key considerations to keep in mind.

A proper warm-up should effectively prepare your muscles and connective tissue for activity. You can use self-myofascial release exercises to ease any tight or sensitive areas. Foam rollers are great for applying pressure to specific areas of your body where you want to increase blood flow and loosen your joints, such as your upper and middle back, which will allow you to twist and rotate with more ease. You can further enhance joint mobility while also gradually warming your body by including dynamic stretches in your warm-up routine. Ideally you should focus on enhancing the range of motion in these four key areas of the body:

1. Ankles

2. Hips

3. Upper back

4. Shoulders

Movements like the Leg Swings (page 96) and Figure 8 (page 98) are great additions to your warm-up routine, as are other functional movements like the Hinge and Reach (page 50) that mimic moves we make in everyday life, like squatting to sit or lunging to climb a flight of stairs. You'll increase your core body temperature, address any struggles you may have with certain movements, improve your range of motion, and reduce your risk of injury. Your dynamic stretches should be intense enough to increase core body temperature gradually but not so intense that you are too wiped out to perform the activity you were warming up for in the first place.

COOLING DOWN

Not only is it important to gradually raise your body temperature and increase your heart rate during the warm-up portion of your workouts, but it is also important to decrease the intensity of activity gradually during the cool-down phase. By taking the time to lower your heart rate and reduce the intensity of your workout, such as by walking or jogging at a slow to moderate pace, you enable the blood to flow back to your heart, as significant amounts of blood also move to your previously working muscles. If you abruptly stop intense exercise, blood may pool in your lower extremities, which could cause you to feel dizzy or even faint. Be careful and give your body the time to transition from intense physical activity back to a state of rest. You also might save yourself from muscle soreness and may even make your muscles more relaxed.

Studies suggest that you benefit most from flexibility exercises when your body is warm, like after you've gone for a bike ride or have done some push-ups. So you are better off performing static stretches during your cool-down. Before you begin stretching in the cool-down phase, you may want to incorporate self-myofascial release to target any particularly tight areas. Foam-rolling exercises will relieve tension and reduce stress in tight areas of your body, such as your glutes and upper back. By following these self-myofascial release exercises with static stretches, such as a Figure 4 (page 92) or Supine Spinal Twist (page 72), you'll increase your flexibility and range of motion, and even improve your posture.

You can vary the length of your cool-down and what's included depending on the type of activity you engaged in; the intensity of those activities; your current fitness level, your personal health, your fitness goals, and the amount of time you have.

BREATHING AND COUNTING

Proper breathing plays an important role while stretching. Slow, rhythmic, mindful breathing—in and out through the nose—will relax you. The pace of your breathing can also keep you in tune with how intensely you should be stretching. If at any point during a stretch you find you are restricting your breathing or holding your breath, this is your cue to reduce the intensity of the stretch so you can breathe freely and naturally.

You can also use your breath to transition in and out of stretches. For example, when you are performing a static stretch, like the Wide-Legged Forward Fold with Chest Expansion (page 108), inhale as you elongate your spine while maintaining proper body alignment, and exhale as you move forward into the fold, holding the end point of the stretch as you breathe freely, in and out through your nose. When you exhale, your diaphragm and the muscles in your chest cavity relax, making the muscles you're stretching relax even further.

Focusing on and refining your breathing also helps you keep track of how long you are holding each stretch without the need to keep your eyes on the clock. Given that the average adult takes 12 to 20 breaths per minute, you can ensure you hold each static stretch for at least 15 seconds by counting five slow and controlled breaths during each stretch repetition. This strategy is easier, more accurate, and more consistent than continuously counting off 15, 30, or 60 seconds while in the middle of a stretch.

PROPS

Stretching is great because it can pretty much be done anywhere, any time, and without expensive equipment. However, depending on the types of stretches you do as part of your flexibility-training routine, you might want to use a few low-cost props and household items to tailor the stretches to meet your personal goals and needs.

When you perform stretches in a seated position, such as the Half Lord of the Fishes (page 88), sit on top of a folded bath towel for additional comfort. The towel also helps position your pelvis correctly and improve your posture.

You can also place a towel beneath your knees for more support in stretches in a kneeling position, such as the Kneeling Lat Stretch (page 78), or roll a towel and place it underneath your lower back when performing stretches like the Head-to-Toe Stretch (page 80).

I find a sturdy chair comes in handy when doing stretches such as the Tibialis Anterior Stretch (page 118), as can a doorway or wall, which can be used as leverage when performing stretches, such as the Assisted Low Lunge (page 110) and the Biceps Stretch (page 56).

You can use a strap or hand towel to stretch safely by applying an appropriate amount of force without pushing your body beyond its limits, for example, when doing the Assisted Supine Hamstring Stretch (page 104). Foam blocks, like the ones used in yoga classes, can also be used to enhance comfort and accessibility in various stretches. Blocks would be a great option for Bound Angle (page 90); place one block beneath each knee for support.

And as mentioned previously, foam rollers are inexpensive, versatile, and worthwhile props for self-myofascial release exercises (see pages 66, 94, and 120).

CHAPTER THREE

YOUR STRETCHING EXPERIENCE

Before you jump right into the stretches, be aware that no two bodies are exactly alike, and you will probably approach your flexibility training in a slightly different way from the next person. In fact, you may even find that your own body feels different from one day to the next.

Everyone Is Different

Because everyone is different, you should always listen to *your body* and home in each day on how the stretches feel today rather than how far you are able to stretch. Remember, your personal stretching routine should be a relaxing and rejuvenating mind-body experience that supports and nourishes your overall health and well-being.

STRETCHING AT EVERY STAGE OF LIFE

While stretching is important for everyone, regardless of age, we all experience changes in our bodies as we grow older. Specifically, for many of us, our muscular strength and flexibility decrease as we age, especially if we are not physically active. In fact, for some, flexibility can decrease by 50 percent in certain areas of the body. As we age, the size and number of muscle fibers in our bodies decrease. Surprisingly, starting at age 30, we lose about a half pound of muscle per year (which equates to five pounds per decade) if we do not regularly complete any resistance training. Because we are losing muscle mass, our muscle fibers are replaced by collagen, which becomes dense and stiff as we grow older, adding to our decreased mobility. Additionally, we lose elastic fibers in our cartilage, ligaments, tendons, and muscles as we age, so our overall flexibility is even further reduced and we are more likely to suffer injuries, such as muscle strains.

But I do have some good news—overwhelming scientific evidence has shown that engaging in regular physical activity, including stretching and range-of-motion exercises, slows physiological changes associated with aging, regardless of your current age or fitness level. Improving your strength and flexibility can increase longevity and enhance overall quality of life!

Myths and Mistakes

You may have come across some of the many myths and misconceptions about flexibility training. As a result, you may be wondering how important stretching really is. Or think that stretching is overly complicated. I'm here to set the record straight on stretching and address mistakes people frequently make when stretching so you do not miss the benefits that it provides.

YOU DON'T HAVE TO BE FLEXIBLE TO STRETCH. Some people assume that stretching is beneficial only for those who are already flexible. The reality is that stretching can improve anyone's flexibility, posture, and body awareness and help alleviate both physical and mental stress. Regardless of how fit you are, include flexibility training as a regular part of your routine. No matter where you start, if you consistently stretch, your flexibility will improve over time and you'll be able to enjoy everyday activities with greater ease.

FOCUS ON ALL THE MAJOR MUSCLES. Many people think the only muscles that need to be stretched are the ones specifically strengthened or targeted during their most recent workout. However, we should focus on all major muscle groups when we stretch. For our bodies to function at their peak, we need to stretch key muscles used during a particular type of activity, and include flexibility exercises for all major muscles, especially those we use every day. For example, after going for a bike ride, we naturally plan to stretch the major muscles we just used, such as our calves, hamstrings, quadriceps, and hip flexors. As part of a complete stretching routine, we should also stretch other muscles we use in our daily activities, such as the back, chest, and shoulders. If we have a balanced, complete approach to stretching, we will feel and function our best.

PROPER FORM IS KEY. Many people assume that to reap the greatest benefit from a stretch, they must move deeply into the stretch, even if they sacrifice good posture and form in the process. Proper body mechanics prevent injury while we reap the intended benefits of each stretch. Avoid rounding your neck and shoulders or back, and hinge at your hips as opposed to your waist when performing any type of forward bend, maintaining an elongated spine. Additionally, strive to bend softly at your knees and elbows to avoid hyperextended or "locking out" the joints.

VARIETY OFFERS BENEFITS (AND BEATS BOREDOM). Your flexibility training can be full of variety. Given the assortment of research-supported strategies for flexibility training, there's no reason your personal stretching routine has to be boring. As seen in chapters 4 through 9, there are many different stretching techniques. This includes stretches inspired by mind-body disciplines like yoga, such as Low Cobra (page 68) and Downward-Facing Dog (page 122), which can provide a fresh approach to improving your flexibility. Listen to music during your stretching workout or add aromatherapy to create an even more relaxing and enjoyable experience.

PAIN DOES NOT MEAN GAIN. When it comes to flexibility training—or any type of physical training for that matter—you don't gain anything by pushing your body to the point of feeling pain. Forcing your body to work beyond its limits not only lessens the potential benefits of stretching, but also significantly increases your risk for injury (and it hurts!). To challenge yourself effectively and safely, stretch only to the point where you feel tightness or slight discomfort—not pain.

SLOW AND STEADY KEEPS YOU SAFE. As noted previously, our muscles are equipped with built-in safety mechanisms to keep us from hurting ourselves. When our muscles detect a change in length, such as during a stretch, a signal is sent to our nervous system that triggers the stretch reflex—the body's attempt to stop the change in muscle length by causing the stretched muscle to contract, or shorten. The more sudden the stretch, the stronger the contraction, which increases tension in the muscle and makes stretching more difficult—which negates the purpose of the stretch itself. It is for this reason that ballistic stretching—a type of dynamic stretching that involves quick bouncing or bobbing motions—is generally not recommended for most adults (with the exception of some well-trained athletes), given the increased risk of injury associated with such rapid movements.

This stretch reflex is also part of the reason it is recommended to hold a static stretch for at least 15 seconds per repetition: This is the length of time that allows the mechanisms within the stretched muscle to become gradually accustomed to the lengthening. This helps minimize the opposing signaling that triggers the reflexive increase in tension—a type of desensitization referred to as stress relaxation. When a stretch is held long enough for this stress relaxation to occur, it allows for a greater range of motion in the joint and a greater stretch of the associated muscle and connective tissue.

A BALANCE OF MOBILITY AND STABILITY. While ensuring the range of uninhibited movement around a joint—known as joint mobility—is important, so, too, is joint *stability*, or the ability to control the position or movement of a joint. While the definition of flexibility, and the purpose of performing stretches, is to improve joint range of motion, for the body to move and function most efficiently and safely, there must be an optimal balance of stability and mobility throughout the entire body. As such, you'll find dynamic stretches in the book, such as Bird-Dog (page 82) and Floor Angels (page 42), designed to enhance stability, especially in key areas like the low back (lumbar spine) and shoulder girdle, while also promoting mobility in the neighboring shoulder and hip joints. This, ultimately, allows for more functional, efficient, and pain-free movement.

IT IS NEVER TOO LATE TO GET STARTED. Stretching offers an assortment of benefits no matter your age or current physical condition. In fact, studies have shown that for individuals over age 50 who pair regular stretching with other forms of physical activity, such as walking or water aerobics, the improvements in flexibility in key areas of the body, such as the hips and shoulders, is significant. This not only helps improve efficiency when performing everyday activities, but can also reduce the likelihood of falls and other injuries like strains and sprains, allowing you to live independently and with enhanced vitality.

Customize Your Routine

Given that every person is different, it's important to understand how to customize your routine to meet your individual needs on any particular day. As such, I encourage you to explore the "Change It Up" feature for each stretch featured in this book. This provides different ways to vary each stretch to create more comfort and support, or add more intensity, depth, or challenge, depending on what you need.

For additional ideas on how to personalize your experience, refer to chapter 14 for tips and strategies for designing your own stretching program.

PART TWO

The
STRETCHES

How to Do the Stretches

While you have countless options when it comes to stretching, in this book, I wanted to provide you with essential static and dynamic stretches for the entire body as well as self-myofascial release techniques for several key areas to help enhance your flexibility and fitness. In this section, you'll find a number of safe and effective stretches that are easy to do at home, at the gym, at work, outdoors, or even on the road while traveling, so you can keep flexibility training and its many benefits a priority.

For each stretch included in this book, I've included easy-to-follow, numbered steps describing how to properly perform the movement, along with information about the benefits of each stretch and the key areas of the body the stretch targets. Make the most out of your stretching routine by using my tips on how to fine tune your form and recommendations on how to vary the stretches using props or other forms of support (such as a table, wall, or chair) to meet your current fitness level, whether that means you want the stretch to be more accessible or more challenging.

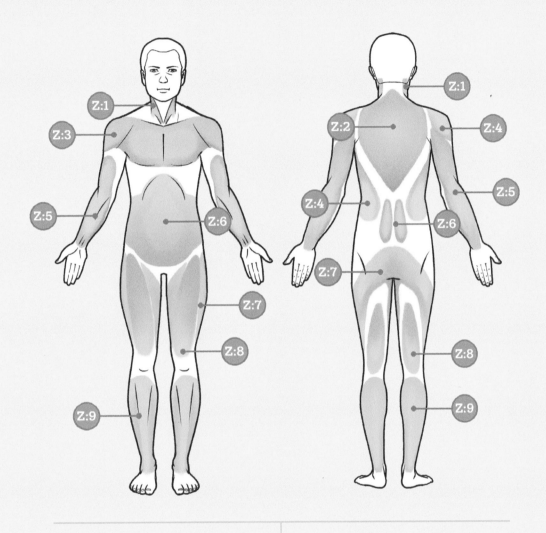

ZONE 1	Neck	ZONE 6	Torso (*rectus abdominis, obliques, transverse abdominis, and erector spinae*)
ZONE 2	Upper back (*trapezius, rhomboids, thoracic spine, scapula*)		
ZONE 3	Front of shoulders (*anterior and middle deltoid*) and chest (*pectorals*)	ZONE 7	Glutes, outer hips (*tensor fascia latae and iliotibial [IT] band*) and inner thighs (*hip adductors*)
ZONE 4	Back of shoulders (*posterior deltoids*) and back (*latissimus dorsi*)	ZONE 8	Hip flexors and thighs (*quadriceps and hamstrings*)
ZONE 5	Upper arms (*biceps brachii and triceps brachii*) and forearms/wrists	ZONE 9	Lower legs/ankles (*anterior tibialis, gastrocnemius and soleus*)

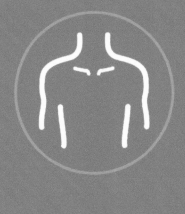

CHAPTER FOUR

NECK, CHEST, and SHOULDERS

THREAD THE NEEDLE

Back of shoulders (*posterior deltoids*),
upper back (*thoracic spine and rhomboids*), and neck

If you find yourself performing overhead activities—from reaching things on a high shelf to throwing a baseball—this stretch is for you. It can also help relieve any pain you may be dealing with because of rotator cuff tendinitis and shoulder bursitis.

COOL DOWN • STATIC

INSTRUCTIONS

1. From a hands-and-knees position, turn your head to the left and slide your right arm along the floor underneath your left arm, positioning your palm to face the ceiling.

2. Keep your hips stacked over your knees, extend your left arm fully in front of your body, and press your right forearm and upper arm (if possible) firmly into the floor. Hold this stretch.

3. Switch sides and repeat.

CHANGE IT UP

- If you want a more accessible version of this stretch, take a seated position and cross one arm across your chest. Using the opposite hand, apply gentle pressure to your upper arm or forearm to pull the crossed arm closer to your body.

- For another variation, assume a standing position facing a wall. Place one arm across your chest and rest your other arm firmly against the wall. Draw the shoulder of the crossed arm closer to the wall for more sensation.

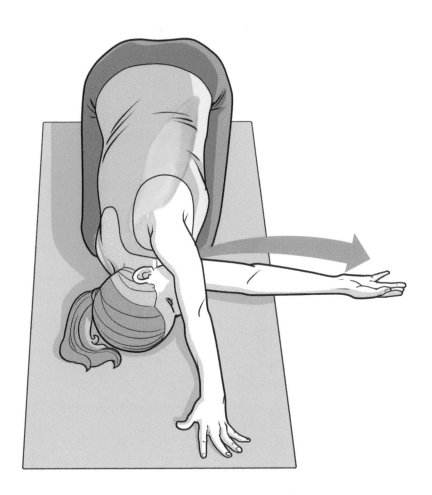

Keep your forearm pressed firmly into the floor and use the
ground as leverage when performing this stretch.

FLOOR ANGELS

Front of shoulders, chest, and back (*latissimus dorsi*)

This dynamic stretch improves range of motion in your shoulder joints, minimizing pain and decreasing the likelihood of shoulder-related injuries.

WARM UP • DYNAMIC

INSTRUCTIONS

1. Lie on your back with your knees bent, feet flat on the floor, arms bent alongside your body, elbows pinned into your sides, and palms facing up.

2. Keeping your arms in contact with the floor, inhale and slide your arms out and over your head until your index fingers touch.

3. As you exhale, slide your arms back down to the starting position, keeping your arms and hands in contact with the floor throughout the movement.

4. Repeat this sequence of movements.

CHANGE IT UP

• To make this stretch more accessible, reduce the range of motion, keeping your elbows slightly more bent as you reach your arms over your head.

• For another variation, perform the movement while standing with your back against a wall.

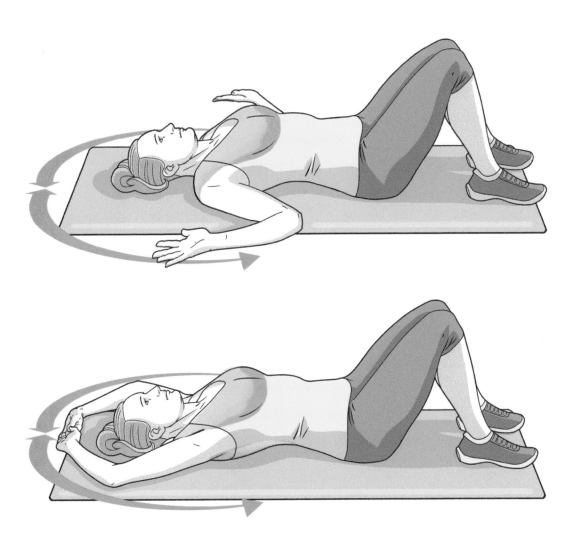

Try to keep your upper arms, forearms, and hands in contact with the surface, or as close as possible, throughout the movement, and avoid arching your lower back as you stretch your arms overhead.

OPEN-HEART STRETCH

Chest, neck, and front of shoulders (*anterior deltoid*)

This simple move stretches your chest, shoulders, and neck muscles that often become tight due to poor posture.

COOL DOWN • STATIC

INSTRUCTIONS

1. While seated, interlace your hands behind the upper back of your head, close to the crown.

2. Gently pull your head forward, guiding your chin toward your chest while keeping your elbows open as wide as possible. Hold this stretch.

CHANGE IT UP

- If you want a slightly less intense neck stretch, perform this stretch in a standing position.

- If you want a slightly more intense neck stretch, draw your chin as low as possible onto your chest.

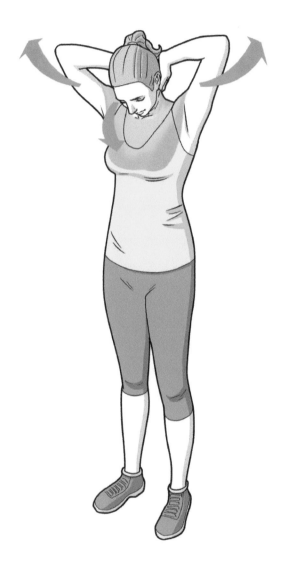

To get the most out of this stretch, avoid rounding your shoulders forward. Instead, focus on engaging the muscles between your shoulder blades to keep your shoulders pulled back and your elbows open wide.

SEATED NECK STRETCH

Neck

This stretch lengthens the neck muscles, which become tight and stiff when you sleep with your head turned to one side, have chronic poor posture, or keep your head in a forward position (often referred to as "tech neck"). In addition to helping alleviate neck pain and discomfort and improving your posture, this stretch may also help minimize headaches.

COOL DOWN • STATIC

INSTRUCTIONS

1. In a seated position, place your left palm on the upper back of your head, just slightly above and behind the right ear.

2. Gently turn your head to the left, then angle your chin down as close to your left shoulder as possible. Hold this stretch.

3. Switch sides and repeat.

CHANGE IT UP

- If you want a slightly less intense stretch, do this stretch in a standing position.

- If you want a slightly more intense stretch, draw your chin as low as possible onto your chest.

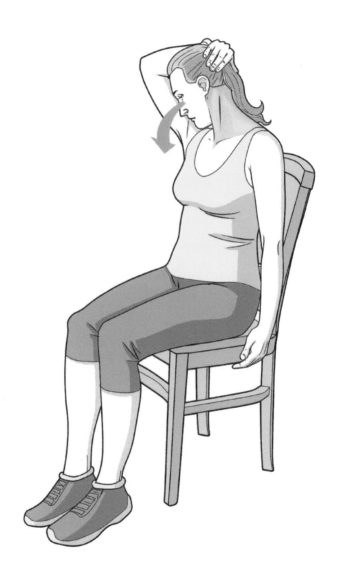

Start by guiding your ear to your shoulder, then point your chin down toward your shoulder. This will make the stretch even more effective at lengthening the neck muscles.

ARM CIRCLES

Shoulders (*front and back*) and upper back

This stretch will give you increased range of motion in your shoulders, while also warming you up for whatever activities may follow.

WARM UP • DYNAMIC

INSTRUCTIONS

1. Stand with your feet hip-width apart. Extend your arms out to your sides at shoulder height, palms facing down.

2. With your elbows extended, slowly begin circling both arms forward simultaneously, starting with a small range of motion (small circles) and gradually making larger circles.

3. Once you complete circling your arms forward, switch directions, making small circles with your arms first and increasing the size of the circles backward to the starting position.

CHANGE IT UP

• For greater ease, keep the circles small and within a range that allows you to remain pain-free. You can also bend your elbows slightly for more comfort.

• For another variation, perform this movement with one arm at a time, noticing any differences between one shoulder and the other.

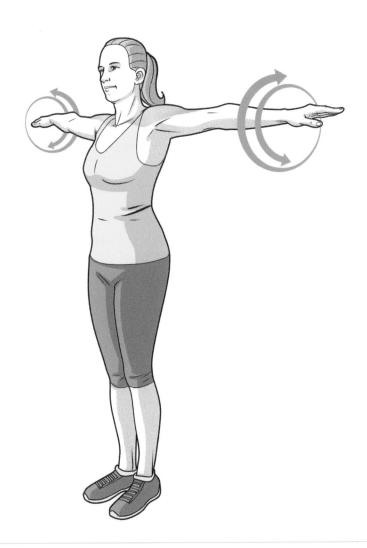

When moving your arms in both directions, start with a smaller range of motion before increasing the size of the circles to explore a larger range of motion.

HINGE AND REACH

Shoulders (*front and back*), back, chest,
upper arms (*biceps and triceps*), and hips (*hip flexors*)

This dynamic stretch is an ideal warm-up move for a wide variety of
everyday tasks and recreational activities, including sports like softball
and tennis that involve swinging and throwing movements.

WARM UP • DYNAMIC

INSTRUCTIONS

1. Stand with your feet hip-width
   apart, arms relaxed alongside
   your body, and palms facing
   each other.

2. Keeping a soft bend in your knees
   and maintaining an elongated
   spine, hinge at the hips, pressing
   your glutes (buttocks) back while
   stretching your arms in front of
   you at shoulder height, palms still
   facing each other.

3. Thrust your hips slightly forward
   and return to a standing position
   while simultaneously swinging
   your arms slightly back behind
   the body.

4. Repeat this sequence.

CHANGE IT UP

- For an alternate version of this
  movement, break this exercise into
  two different dynamic stretches.
  Focus first on swinging your arms
  front and back, and then work
  exclusively on the hip hinge.

- For another variation, swap the
  hip-hinging movement for a half
  squat, bending your knees as you
  shift your hips back and down.

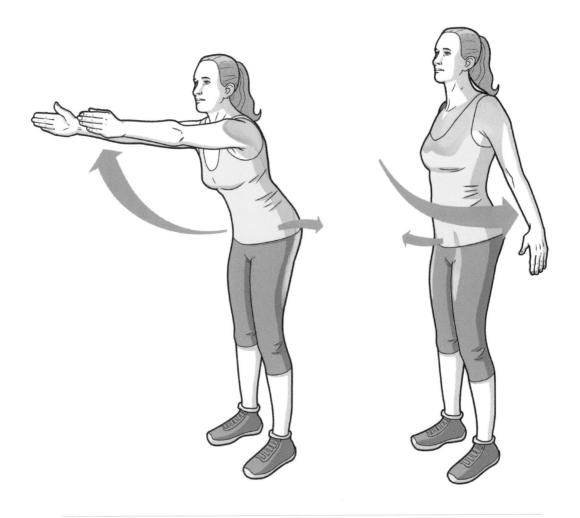

This dynamic stretch is a warm-up exercise. Therefore, it's important to go through the movements at a slow, controlled pace to allow your body to prepare gradually for the activity to follow.

REVERSE TABLETOP

Chest, neck, and hips (*hip flexors*)

This move stretches various muscles, such as the pectorals and hip flexors. These muscles can become tight and stiff from sitting for long periods of time, whether working at a desk or driving a car.

COOL DOWN • STATIC

INSTRUCTIONS

1. In a seated position with your knees bent and feet flat on the floor, place your palms directly behind your body with your fingers pointed toward your backside.

2. Inhale while gently pressing into your hands and your feet to lift your glutes (buttocks) off the floor, extending your hips toward the ceiling.

3. Exhale and gently draw your shoulder blades toward each other to open your chest toward the ceiling while carefully lowering your head back and tilting your chin up. Hold this stretch.

CHANGE IT UP

• To vary this stretch, lie on your back with your knees bent, feet flat on the floor, arms at your sides. Press into your hands and feet to lift your glutes (buttocks) off the mat for a bridge pose. To stretch your chest and shoulders, shimmy your arms underneath your body and interlace your fingers while holding this raised position, lifting your chest and hips toward the ceiling.

• For a more intense stretch, extend your legs fully and lift your hips, rooting the soles of your feet into the ground for a reverse plank position.

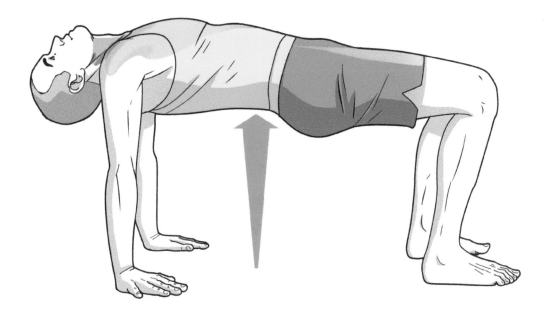

Because of the sheer weight of your head, lower your head back in a slow and controlled fashion, gradually tilting your chin toward the ceiling to avoid placing undue stress on your neck.

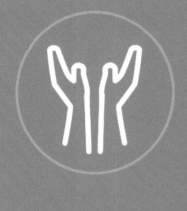

CHAPTER FIVE

ARMS, HANDS, and WRISTS

BICEPS STRETCH

Upper arms (*biceps*) and forearms/wrists

This stretch is perfect for stretching the key muscles that flex the elbows. It's ideal if you spend many hours on the phone, typing on a keyboard, lifting heavy boxes, or suffer from carpal tunnel syndrome or golfer's elbow.

COOL DOWN • STATIC

INSTRUCTIONS

1. Stand with your hips and shoulders parallel to a wall. Place your right palm against the surface (fingers pointing to the right, thumb pointing up) with your arm fully extended at shoulder height. Keep your left arm relaxed at your side.

2. Keeping your palm in contact with the wall, pivot on your feet to rotate your body to the left, assuming a split-stance position—with your left foot forward and right foot back. Plant both feet firmly as you rotate your hip and shoulder away from the wall. Hold this stretch.

3. Switch sides and repeat.

CHANGE IT UP

- If you want to decrease the intensity of this stretch, keep a slight bend in the elbow of your extended arm.

- To increase the intensity of the stretch, press your hand firmly into the wall and shift your chest slightly forward to deepen the stretch.

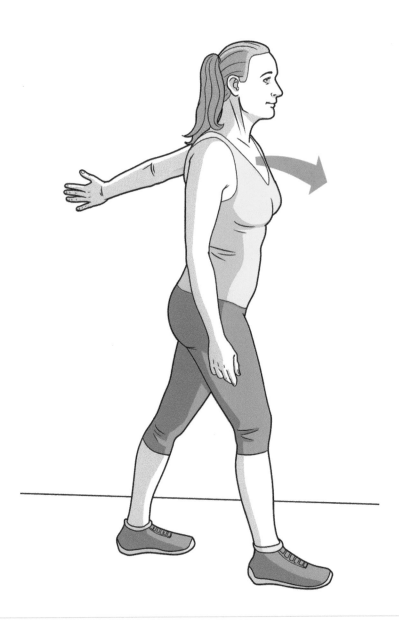

While you should, ideally, position your arm at shoulder height, you can still reap the benefits of this stretch by placing your arm slightly lower on the wall.

OVERHEAD TRICEPS STRETCH

Upper arms (*triceps*)

You use your triceps every time you "push" something, from dumbbell shoulder presses and push-ups at the gym to closing your car door and propping yourself up from a lying to a seated position. Be sure to stretch this important muscle to avoid injury.

COOL DOWN • STATIC

INSTRUCTIONS

1. Stand with your feet hip-width apart. Extend your right arm over your head, bending at the elbow and turning your palm to touch the center of your upper back.

2. Keeping your right elbow close to your right ear, place your left hand on top of your right elbow and gently apply pressure, pushing your right palm farther down your back. Hold this stretch.

3. Switch sides and repeat.

CHANGE IT UP

- If you have trouble with your balance, perform this stretch while seated.

- To vary the sensation of this stretch, simultaneously pull your elbow closer to your ear while applying downward pressure on your arm.

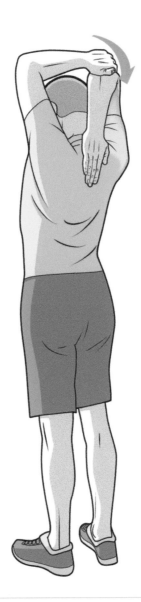

Keep your back straight and avoid curling your neck when doing this stretch.

WRIST-EXTENSOR STRETCH

Forearms/wrists

Tennis players and gym-goers: Include this stretch in your flexibility training. It's perfect for stretching those muscles that act on the wrists and may relieve your tennis elbow!

COOL DOWN • STATIC

INSTRUCTIONS

1. Stand with your feet hip-width apart. Extend your right arm in front of your body at shoulder height, palm facing down.

2. Keeping your palm down and elbow extended, point your right fingers toward the floor. Press your left hand against the knuckles of your right hand, drawing your fingers closer to your body. Hold this stretch.

3. Switch sides and repeat.

CHANGE IT UP

• For even more comfort and support, perform this stretch in a seated position at your desk.

• For a variation of this stretch, assume a kneeling position with your palms on the floor and your fingers pointed toward your body. Shift your hips slightly back toward your heels while keeping both palms firmly planted on the ground, creating your desired level of sensation.

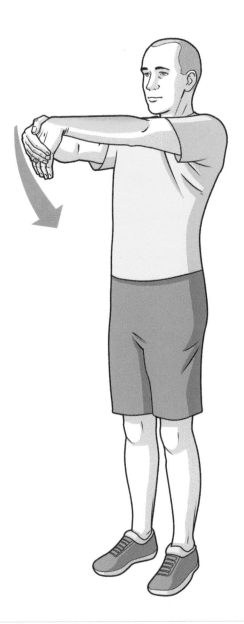

When you do this stretch, gently draw your fingers toward you so you don't cause any pain in your fingers or wrist.

WRIST-FLEXOR STRETCH

Forearms/wrists

After spending long periods of time with your wrists in a flexed position, such as when typing or talking on the phone, this stretch will help alleviate any discomfort.

COOL DOWN • STATIC

INSTRUCTIONS

1. Stand with your feet hip-width apart. Interlace your fingers and flip your palms to face away from your body.

2. Raise your arms to shoulder height and extend your elbows, while simultaneously pushing your palms away from your body. Hold this stretch.

CHANGE IT UP

- For even more comfort and support, perform this stretch in a seated position at your desk.

- To add a little variety to this move and provide some stretch for your back and forearms, extend your arms over your head with your palms facing the ceiling.

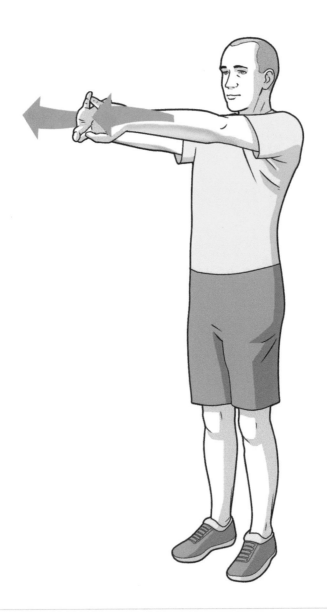

Keep your elbows extended and focus on pushing your palms away from your body to maximize this stretch.

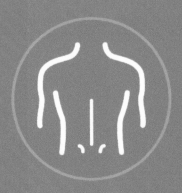

CHAPTER SIX

BACK and TORSO

SELF-MYOFASCIAL RELEASE FOR MID AND UPPER BACK

Upper back (*thoracic spine*)

This technique enhances mobility in your thoracic spine, a key series of joints in the mid and upper back that we use when we perform any rotational movements, such as swinging a tennis racket or shoveling snow. This exercise requires a foam roller.

WARM UP • COOL DOWN • PROP (FOAM ROLLER)

INSTRUCTIONS

1. Sit on the ground with your knees bent and feet on the floor. Place a foam roller behind your back near your shoulder blades.

2. Cross your arms over your chest and roll your body back so the middle of your back ends up on top of the foam roller.

3. Move your body back and forth on the foam roller, using small (2- to 6-inch) continuous movements over your mid and upper back, applying gentle pressure to any tender areas where you feel discomfort.

CHANGE IT UP

- If you have a particularly tender spot on your back, apply pressure near, but not directly over, the area and hold for up to 60 seconds.

- To enhance the feeling of release you get from this move, position your foam roller directly over the tender area you are targeting and apply pressure, holding the position for up to 30 seconds.

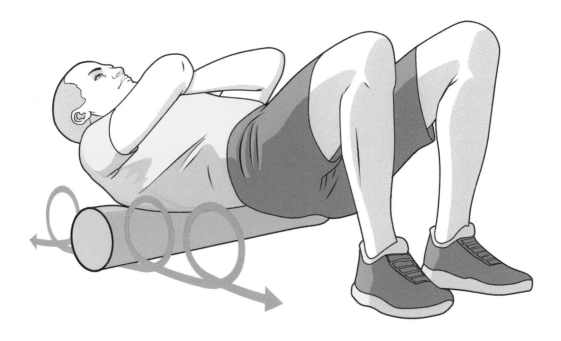

In addition to moving back and forth, allow your spine to drape over the foam roller, almost as if you were performing subtle mini crunches. This gentle arching of your upper back will help increase its extension, which can make your shoulders feel less restricted when you lift your arms overhead to put away groceries or dishes in high cabinets.

LOW COBRA

Torso (*abdominals*)

Inspired by yoga, this move stretches your abdominal muscles and is a great counterbalance to spending many hours seated at a desk or driving a car, where your upper back may be in a rounded position and cause lower-back pain. Also, by stretching your abdominal muscles, you improve your breathing, which can become restricted if abdominal muscles are tight.

COOL DOWN • STATIC

INSTRUCTIONS

1. Lie on your stomach with your elbows bent and your hands below your shoulders. Stretch out your legs, hip-width apart, resting the tops of your feet on the floor.

2. Keep your palms and the tops of your feet pressed into the floor. Inhale as you slide your chest slightly forward and lift it off the floor. Engage your glutes (buttocks) and extend your elbows slightly while keeping your arms close to your body. Hold this position.

3. Exhale as you lower your chest back to the floor.

CHANGE IT UP

- For an easier stretch that still targets the same muscles, lie on your back with a rolled towel beneath the small of your back. This support will help minimize the pressure placed on your spine.

- To increase the intensity of this stretch, extend your elbows fully and lift your chest, belly, and thighs off the floor, coming into upward-facing dog.

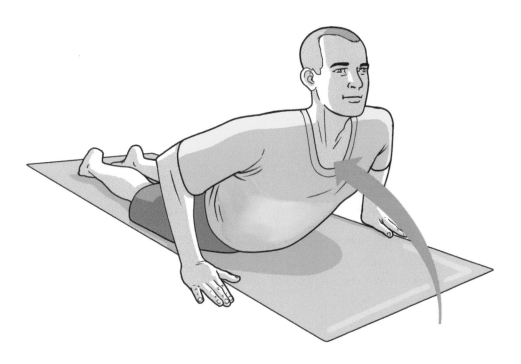

To move into this stretch safely, start by sliding your chest slightly forward before lifting it off the floor. In addition, engaging your glutes when arching your spine relieves some of the stress on your lower back.

CAT-COW

Back (*thoracic spine*), torso (*abdominals*), ankles, and neck

This dynamic motion exercise helps loosen your upper back and gets you ready to tackle everyday tasks, while also effectively warming you up for various activities, like dancing, swimming, and cycling.

WARM UP • DYNAMIC

INSTRUCTIONS

1. Begin in a hands-and-knees position, with your wrists aligned below your shoulders and your knees aligned below your hips. Keep your spine extended and your toes tucked under.

2. Inhale, relax your belly so it moves toward the floor, and gently arch your back, tilting your tailbone and chin toward the ceiling.

3. Exhale, gently round your spine, draw your chin toward your chest, and untuck your toes, placing the tops of your feet on the floor.

4. Repeat this sequence of movements.

CHANGE IT UP

- To make this move more accessible, do it in a seated position, either on the floor or in a chair. Place your palms on top of your thighs and gently round and arch your back.

- To modify this movement, round your spine as you exhale while simultaneously shifting your hips back toward your heels. When you inhale, shift your weight forward and return to all fours before softening your belly and arching your spine to continue the sequence.

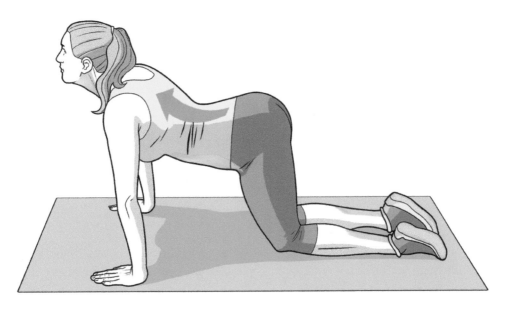

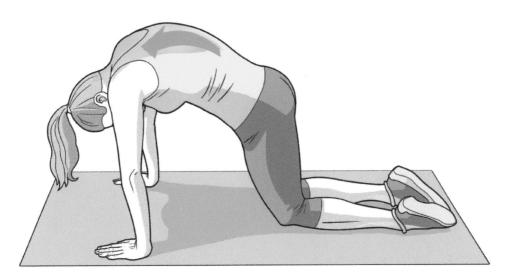

With this exercise, you are moving rather than staying static, so focus more on the movement itself rather than on deepening the stretch.

SUPINE SPINAL TWIST

Back, torso, and outer hips

This gentle twist relieves tension in your spine by stretching the muscles in your back. It also helps reduce any feelings of stress and anxiety you may have, making this a welcome stretch at the end of a busy day.

COOL DOWN • STATIC

INSTRUCTIONS

1. While lying on your back with your knees bent and feet flat, stretch your left leg along the floor, keeping a slight bend in the knee.

2. Inhale, lift your right foot, and, with your hands, draw your right knee toward your chest.

3. Exhale, extend your right arm, palm facing up, out to your right side. With your left hand, gently guide your right knee across your body to fall outside your left hip.

4. Turn your head to look toward your right hand. Hold this stretch.

5. Switch sides and repeat.

CHANGE IT UP

- For more support, place a foam block on the outside of your hip and rest your bent knee on top of the block.

- To vary the sensation, scoot your hips slightly toward the direction of your outstretched arm and use your other hand as leverage on your bent knee to deepen the rotation and stretch.

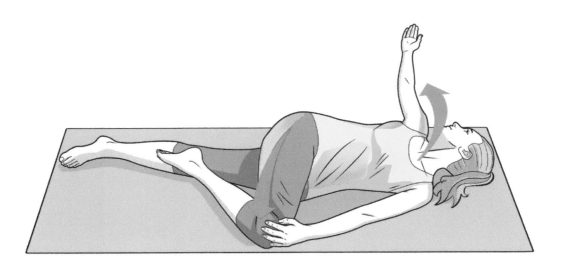

Keep both shoulders in contact with the floor, or as close as you can, when you perform this twist.

STANDING CRESCENT MOON

Torso (*obliques and quadratus lumborum*)

This stretch focuses on lateral flexion, or side-to-side movement of the spine, an important action that can help reduce incidents of lower-back pain while improving your posture.

COOL DOWN • STATIC

INSTRUCTIONS

1. Stand with your feet hip-width apart, arms at your sides.

2. Inhale, sweeping your left arm toward the ceiling with your palm facing to the right.

3. Exhale, reach your left fingertips up and over toward your right side, leaning your torso to the right to stretch the left side of your body. Hold this stretch.

4. Switch sides and repeat.

CHANGE IT UP

- For greater support, perform this stretch seated on the edge of a chair with your feet flat on the floor, one arm relaxed at your side or resting on your thigh if you are using a chair with arms.

- For a deeper stretch, extend both arms up and overhead with palms pressed together.

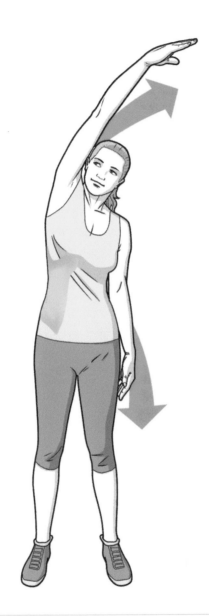

To stretch the side of your body effectively, focus first on reaching your extended arm up before reaching over to the other side.

BEAR HUG

Back of shoulders, back (*latissimus dorsi*), and upper back (*rhomboids and trapezius*)

If you experience pain in your shoulders, particularly around your shoulder blades, because of poor posture, this stretch will help. It can also be of benefit if you suffer from shoulder issues such as bursitis or frozen shoulder. Additionally, this stretch can make it easier for you to perform household duties that require reaching overhead.

COOL DOWN • STATIC

INSTRUCTIONS

1. Stand with your feet hip-width apart, arms open wide.

2. Cross one arm over the other at your elbows, reaching your hands over your opposite shoulders as if giving yourself a hug.

3. Gently draw the shoulders forward. Hold this stretch.

CHANGE IT UP

- If it is too difficult to reach your shoulders, perform this stretch by grasping the upper portion of the opposite arm instead of your shoulder, drawing your forearms parallel with each other as you gently pull your shoulders forward.

- For a more intense stretch, use a doorway: Cross one arm in front of your body at shoulder height. Point your thumb down and extend your elbow while grabbing hold of the doorjamb. Rotate your body gently in the opposite direction to create your desired level of stretch. Repeat on the other side.

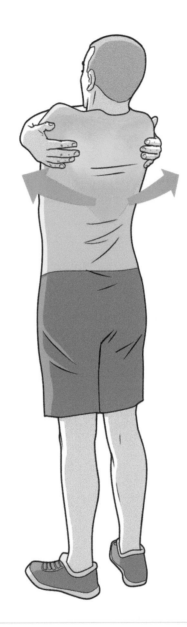

Each time you repeat this stretch, alternate crossing your arms and note whether one side feels more comfortable than the other.

KNEELING LAT STRETCH

Back (*latissimus dorsi*)

This stretch targets your latissimus dorsi, the large muscle of your back, and helps make everyday activities that involve reaching your arms overhead, such as taking something off a high shelf, as well as recreational activities like swimming, easier to perform. Additionally, when you stretch this key muscle, you help prevent shoulder pain and discomfort, including rotator cuff injuries.

COOL DOWN • STATIC • PROP (BLANKET OR TOWEL)

INSTRUCTIONS

1. Start in a kneeling position, facing the seat of a chair or a couch, and rest your knees, hip-width apart, on a folded blanket or towel for additional comfort.

2. Keep your spine extended and bend at your hips to create a 90-degree angle with your body as you place your forearms, palms facing each other, on top of the seat in front of you. Hold this stretch.

CHANGE IT UP

- To make this stretch more accessible, start in a standing position and use a table or countertop instead of a chair. Keep your palms down to reduce the stretch.

- To deepen the stretch, turn your palms up to the ceiling or join them together and bend your elbows.

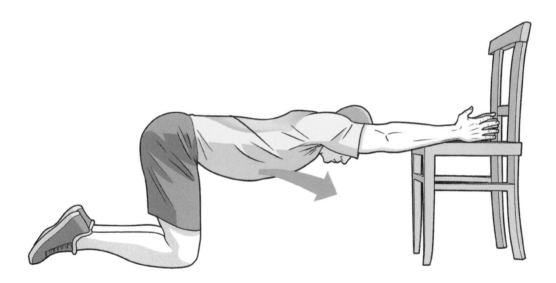

As you bend forward, keep your hips stacked over your knees and place your elbows close to the edge of the seat while actively outstretching your arms.

HEAD-TO-TOE STRETCH

Torso (*abdominals*), back (*latissimus dorsi*), and lower legs/ankles (*tibialis anterior*)

This full-body stretch stretches your abdominal muscles, which can become tight as a result of poor posture and cause lower-back pain. Using the towel in this exercise helps reduce any undue pressure on your spine. Reaching your arms overhead while pointing your toes stretches your back and shins.

COOL DOWN • STATIC • PROP (TOWEL)

INSTRUCTIONS

1. From a seated position with your knees bent and feet flat on the floor, place a small rolled towel beneath the small of your back. Recline into a lying position, stretching out your legs along the floor.

2. Inhale, stretch your arms over your head, palms facing the ceiling, allowing your arms and hands to touch the floor or draw as close to the floor as possible while keeping your back in contact with the towel. At the same time, point your toes away from your body. Keep your glutes (buttocks), upper back, and the back of your head in contact with the floor at all times. Hold this stretch.

CHANGE IT UP

- To support your lower back even more, keep your knees bent with your feet flat on the floor.

- For a more intense and deeper stretch, roll the towel into a slightly larger size to increase the stretch in your abs.

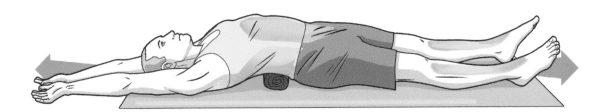

When performing this stretch, gently squeeze your buttocks to minimize the stress placed on your lower back. Keep your glutes, upper back, and the back of your head in contact with the floor at all times.

BIRD-DOG

Torso

This dynamic motion exercise builds stability in your lumbar spine, thereby reducing your risk of lower-back pain.

WARM UP • DYNAMIC

INSTRUCTIONS

1. Begin in a hands-and-knees position with your wrists aligned below your shoulders and knees below your hips; your fingers should point forward.

2. Tuck your right toes under and extend your right leg behind you. Slowly lift your leg off the floor, raising it no higher than hip height.

3. Brace your core gently so you maintain an elongated spine. Slowly reach your left arm forward, no higher than shoulder height, and turn your palm to face inward while pointing your thumb toward the ceiling. Hold this extended position for no more than 7 to 8 seconds, keeping your hips and shoulders level.

4. Return to the starting position and repeat the movement on your opposite side.

CHANGE IT UP

- For greater ease, break this exercise down into two different movements. Focus first on extending your leg behind you, either keeping your toes on the ground or lifting them. Return to the starting position with both knees on the ground, before extending your opposite arm forward.

- For a variation, perform several repetitions (3 or 4) with your right leg/left arm, lowering your limbs just until they brush the floor between lifts. Switch sides and repeat this exercise with your opposite arm and leg (left leg/ right arm).

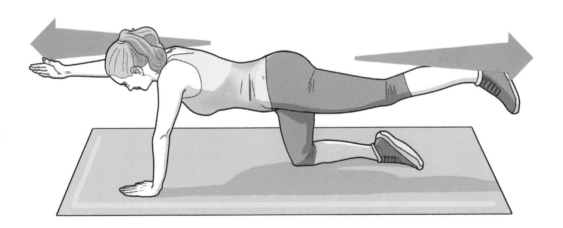

You're more likely to build endurance by increasing the number of repetitions you do as opposed to holding your arm and leg extended for a longer period time. Therefore, hold the range of motion for no more than 7 to 8 seconds and avoid shifting your weight when alternating sides.

QUADRUPED ROTATIONS

Upper back (*thoracic spine*)

This dynamic stretch increases your range of motion in your upper back, helpful for so many everyday movements—from reaching across your body to put on a seat belt to swinging a golf club.

WARM UP • DYNAMIC

INSTRUCTIONS

1. Begin in a hands-and-knees position with your knees aligned below your hips and your wrists below your shoulders.

2. Draw your left fingertips behind your left ear, keeping your elbow bent and open to the side of your body.

3. Rotate your torso to your left, drawing your left elbow to point toward the ceiling.

4. Reverse the movement, returning your torso to your starting position parallel with the floor while crossing your left elbow toward your right arm. Continue this movement.

5. Switch sides and repeat.

CHANGE IT UP

- If your wrists or knees bother you when you are in a hands-and-knees position, try this dynamic stretch while seated, with both sets of fingers behind your ears and your elbows out wide.

- For a different variation, perform this rotational movement in a high-kneeling position with both sets of fingers behind your ears and your elbows wide. As you rotate in one direction, dip one elbow toward the ground, followed by the other, and twist a little bit more in the same direction to increase your range of motion.

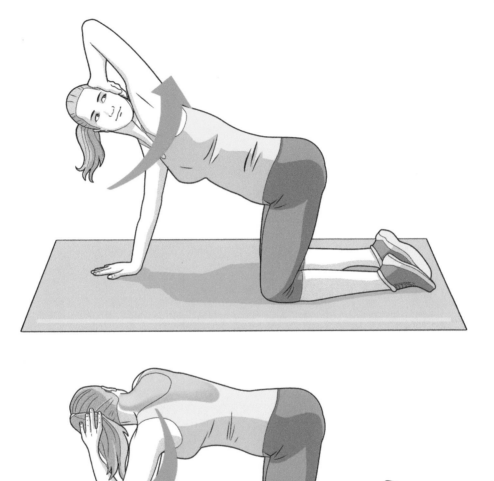

To reduce pressure on your spine, visualize rotating your entire torso, including your head and neck, as one unit when moving in each direction, twisting from your upper back in a controlled fashion.

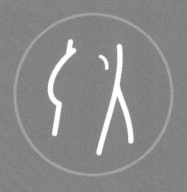

CHAPTER SEVEN

HIPS and GLUTES

HALF LORD OF THE FISHES

Outer hips, glutes, and torso (*erector spinae*)

This stretch is beneficial if you suffer from lower-back and hip pain, including sciatica.

COOL DOWN • STATIC

INSTRUCTIONS

1. Sit on the floor with your legs out-stretched in front of you. Bend your right knee and step your right foot over your left thigh, planting your right foot on the floor outside your left knee.

2. Place your right hand behind your right hip with your fingers pointed away from your body. Inhale and lift your left arm toward the ceiling while lengthening your spine.

3. Exhale, gently rotate your torso to the right, hugging your right knee with your left arm or hooking your left elbow outside your right knee. Gaze over your right shoulder, if you can manage it. Hold this stretch.

4. Switch sides and repeat.

CHANGE IT UP

- For more support and comfort, sit on a folded blanket, towel, or foam block.

- For a more intense stretch, bend your extended leg, folding your heel in toward your opposite glute.

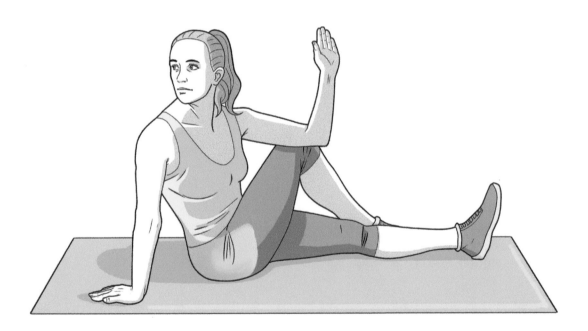

Maintain length in your spine when performing this stretch and allow your head to turn to face the same direction you are twisting.

BOUND ANGLE

Inner thighs (*hip adductors*), back (*erector spinae*)

This stretch for your inner thighs is beneficial if you participate in recreational activities like cross-country skiing or dancing.

COOL DOWN • STATIC

INSTRUCTIONS

1. Sit on the floor with your knees bent and draw the soles of your feet together. Let your knees release away from each other.

2. Place your hands on the tops of your feet or just above your ankles while keeping the outer edges of your feet in contact with the floor. Inhale and maintain length in your spine.

3. Exhale, lean slightly forward, draw your chest toward your heels, and press your elbows gently into your thighs. Hold for 3 to 5 breaths.

CHANGE IT UP

- Place a foam block or rolled towel beneath each knee for additional support.

- To deepen the stretch, position your heels closer to your tailbone.

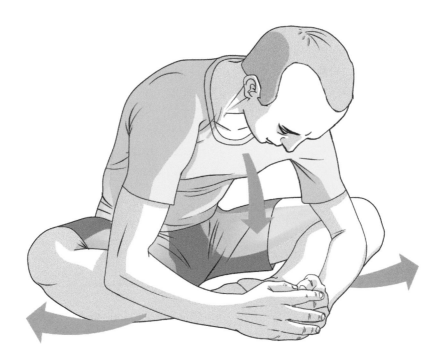

Leaning your body forward deepens the stretch in the inner thigh muscles while also stretching the muscles of your lower back.

FIGURE 4

Outer hips and glutes

This stretch for the outer hips is of benefit if you walk, run, hike, or bike regularly.

COOL DOWN • STATIC

INSTRUCTIONS

1. Lie on your back with your knees bent, feet flat on the floor. Lift your right foot, crossing your right ankle to your left knee as your right knee opens to the right.

2. Keep your head, neck, and shoulders in contact with the floor and lift your left foot off the ground, keeping your left knee bent.

3. Thread your right arm through the space between your legs and reach your left arm around your left leg to interlace your hands behind your left thigh. Guide your left knee toward your chest and hold this stretch.

4. Slowly unthread your arms and release your legs to return to the starting position.

5. Switch sides and repeat.

CHANGE IT UP

- Keep one knee bent with one foot on the floor and your arms relaxed at your sides for an easier stretch.

- Pull your knee closer toward your chest while using your elbow to nudge your opposite knee farther open to the side for a deeper stretch.

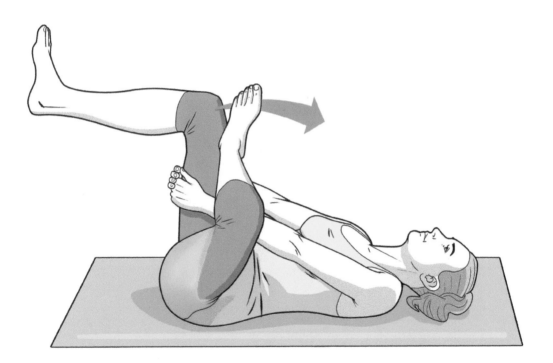

Draw both sets of toes toward your shins to help stabilize your knees while you work through this stretch.

Figure 4   93

SELF-MYOFASCIAL RELEASE FOR GLUTES

Outer hips and glutes

This move targets tight, restricted areas of your fascia (see page 22) as well as the underlying glutes. If you play sports like golf or tennis, where you make a lot of repetitive movements in one direction, resulting in a muscle imbalance, include this move in your training routine. You will need a foam roller.

WARM UP • COOL DOWN • PROP (FOAM ROLLER)

INSTRUCTIONS

1. Sitting on a foam roller with your knees bent and your feet on the floor, place your right hand on the ground with your fingers angled away from your body directly behind the foam roller.

2. Keep your left leg bent, extend your right leg fully, and angle your body slightly, shifting your weight to your right so the roller is positioned underneath your backside.

3. Roll your body back and forth on the foam roller using small (2- to 6-inch) continuous movements, applying gentle pressure to any tender areas.

4. Switch sides and repeat.

CHANGE IT UP

- If you have a particularly tender spot in your glutes, apply pressure near, but not directly over, the area and hold for up to 60 seconds.

- To deepen the release of a sore or tender spot, position the foam roller directly over the area and apply pressure, holding for up to 30 seconds.

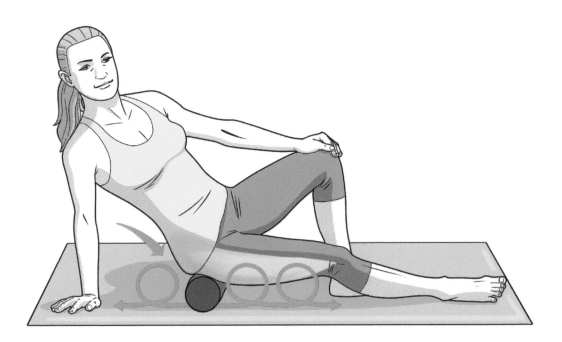

You can control the intensity of any discomfort by using more or less pressure, depending on your tolerance level. To achieve an even greater release of tension, breathe slowly and deeply through your nose, which helps you feel more relaxed.

LEG SWINGS

Outer hips (*tensor fasciae latae*), glutes,
thighs (*quadriceps and hamstrings*), and hip flexors

This is a great dynamic warm-up to do before tackling everyday activities or engaging in high-intensity workouts, such as running, hiking, or cycling.

WARM UP • DYNAMIC • PROP (WALL OR CHAIR, IF NEEDED)

INSTRUCTIONS

1. Stand with your feet slightly parted and your hands resting on your hips.

2. Shift your weight to your left foot, bending your right knee slightly while lifting your right heel.

3. Keeping your right knee softly bent, actively swing your right leg forward and backward, allowing your right knee to naturally bend and extend throughout the movement, all while keeping your back straight. Continue this movement.

4. Switch sides and repeat.

CHANGE IT UP

• If you need assistance with balance, use a wall or the back of a sturdy chair for support.

• To deepen the stretch, increase the range of motion when you swing your leg forward and back while keeping your torso in an upright position and your back straight.

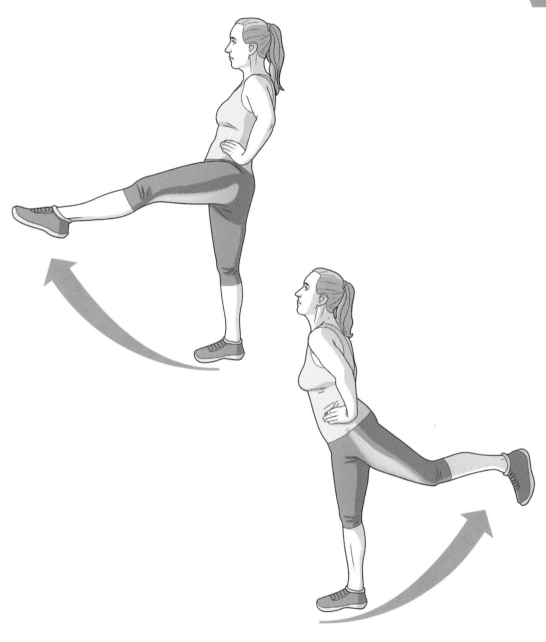

Perform this movement at a controlled, rhythmic tempo. When using dynamic stretches to warm up, start with front-to-back movements, such as this one, before switching to side-to-side or rotational moves.

FIGURE 8

Outer hip, glutes, inner thighs, and ankles

This active stretch targets your hip's deep muscles and is a great prep for activities that require quick changes in speed and direction, like tennis and dancing. Also, if you have arthritis, you may ease some of the stiffness and pain associated with the condition when you perform these hip circles.

WARM UP • DYNAMIC • PROP (WALL OR CHAIR)

INSTRUCTIONS

1. Stand facing a wall, doorframe, or the back of a sturdy chair. Fully extend your arms and place both hands on the wall or chair.

2. Shift your weight to your left foot. Bend your right knee slightly while lifting your right heel, keeping your toes on the floor.

3. With your right knee bent, trace a figure 8 pattern on the floor with your toes, extending your right hip and knee and then bringing them in closer to you in a fluid motion. Continue this movement.

4. Switch sides and repeat.

CHANGE IT UP

• For more support, perform this stretch on your hands and knees rather than standing.

• To add a little more challenge to this exercise, perform this movement away from a wall, keeping your hands on your hips to work on your balance.

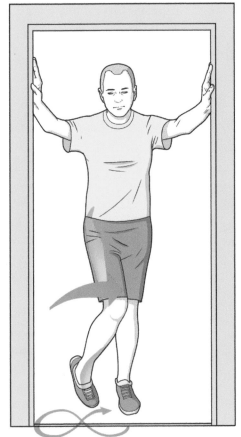
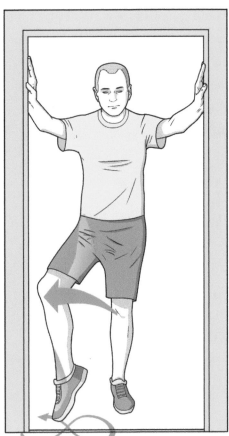

For your safety, keep this move within your comfortable range of motion and gradually increase the size of the circles as you grow more comfortable. Remember to complete this stretch in a smooth, fluid manner.

Figure 8   99

SIDE-TO-SIDE STANDING DIAGONALS

Inner thighs, outer hips, shoulders (*front and back*), and torso

To loosen your hips and improve your knee stability, add this dynamic stretch to your repertoire. Lateral movements improve hip mobility, and cross-body arm movements make your shoulders feel less restricted and can reduce the likelihood of rotator cuff injury.

WARM UP • DYNAMIC

INSTRUCTIONS

1. Stand with your feet together. Raise your right arm and a loose fist out and away from your body, toward the ceiling, at a 45-degree angle.

2. Step your right foot out 1 to 2 feet to your right, turning your body at the hips and bending your right knee to go into a side lunge. At the same time, cross your right arm in front of your body with your elbow bent and your hand in front of your left hip, your right forearm parallel to your belly.

3. Gently push off your right foot, returning back to your starting position with your feet together and your right arm raised. Continue this movement.

4. Switch sides and repeat.

CHANGE IT UP

- For greater ease, break the movement down into two different parts. Focus first on the side-to-side lunging movement with your hands on your hips; then on rotating at the hips while standing, keeping your arms in a stationary position.

- To test your coordination, start this stretch with both arms extended to form a *V* shape. Alternate sides, lunging to your left and right while alternating which arm you cross for each repetition.

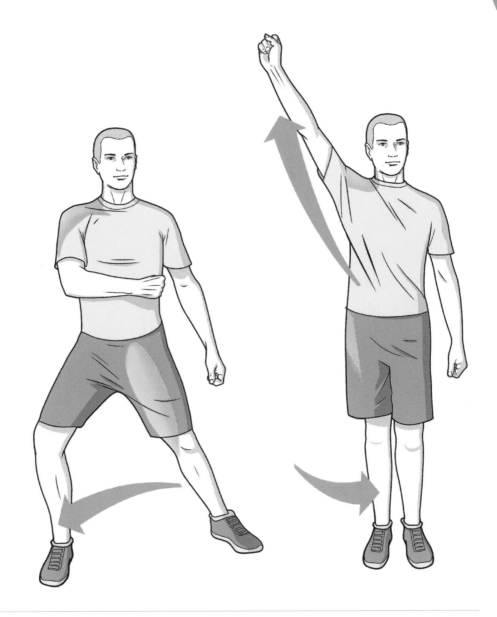

Avoid stepping too far out to your side during the lunge and keep the knee of the bent leg in line with the second toe of that foot to avoid straining your knee or hip.

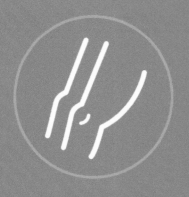

CHAPTER EIGHT

KNEES and THIGHS

ASSISTED SUPINE HAMSTRING STRETCH

Thighs (*hamstrings*) and lower legs/ankles (*gastrocnemius and soleus*)

The hamstrings can become tight after activities like running and hiking. It is important to stretch your hamstrings to avoid and alleviate lower-back pain. You will need a strap for this.

COOL DOWN • STATIC • PROP (STRAP)

INSTRUCTIONS

1. Lie on your back with your knees bent, feet flat on the floor. Draw your right knee toward your chest, looping the strap around the sole of your right foot. Hold one end of the strap in each hand with your palms facing each other.

2. Extend your left leg out in front of you on the floor while extending your right leg up, pressing your right heel toward the ceiling to draw your leg as perpendicular to the floor as possible.

3. Keep the back of your head and shoulders on the ground. Apply gentle pressure to your right foot using the strap, bending your elbows and drawing your toes toward your shin. Hold this stretch.

4. Switch sides and repeat.

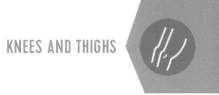
CHANGE IT UP

- For more support, ditch the strap and perform this stretch in a doorway instead, resting your extended leg against the door frame. You can change the deepness of the stretch by positioning your buttocks closer to or farther from the door frame.

- For a deeper stretch, perform this as a PNF stretch (see page 23), pressing your foot against the strap to resist the stretch, contracting your hamstrings for 3 to 6 seconds before using the strap to bring your knee closer toward your body, holding it for 15 to 30 seconds.

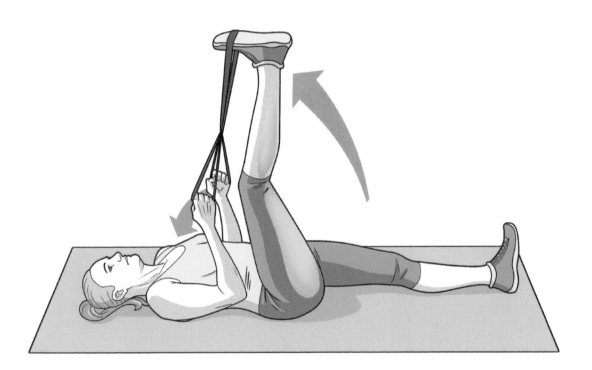

Drawing the toes toward your shin while doing this hamstring stretch also gives your calf muscles a good stretch.

SUPPORTED STANDING QUADRICEPS STRETCH

Thighs (*quadriceps*) and hip flexors

This stretch focuses on your quads, or quadriceps (the muscles that make up the front of your thighs), which you use daily for such activities as walking, climbing stairs, and standing.

COOL DOWN • STATIC • PROP (WALL OR CHAIR; TOWEL OR STRAP)

INSTRUCTIONS

1. Stand with your feet hip-width apart, parallel to a wall or the back of a sturdy chair. Place your right hand on the surface for support.

2. Shift your weight to your right foot and bend your left knee, pulling your heel toward your glutes and reaching your left hand behind to grasp the top of your left foot or ankle.

3. Keep your left knee close to and in line with your right knee. Shift your hips slightly forward. Hold this stretch.

4. Switch sides and repeat.

CHANGE IT UP

- For a more accessible support, lie on your side, keeping your bottom leg extended as you bend your top leg to stretch your thigh. If you need an easier version of this stretch, use a towel or strap to draw the heel of your top leg back toward your glutes (buttocks).

- To test your balance, do this stretch away from the wall, keeping your free hand on your hip.

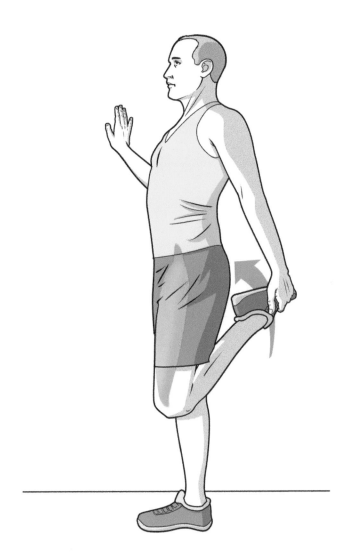

When doing this stretch, point your knee down toward the ground so your thigh is perpendicular with the floor and your knees are in line with each other.

WIDE-LEGGED FORWARD FOLD WITH CHEST EXPANSION

Thighs (*hamstrings*), inner thighs (*certain hip adductors*), torso (*erector spinae*), chest, and front of shoulders

This yoga-inspired stretch targets major muscles of your upper and lower body, with primary attention on the hamstrings, a muscle group that can become tight when you walk, hike, run, and bike, among other activities. The use of a strap helps stretch tight muscles in your chest and shoulders from all the long hours we spend typing or driving.

COOL DOWN • STATIC • PROP (STRAP)

INSTRUCTIONS

1. Stand with your feet wide, about 3 to 4 feet apart, and parallel to each other, knees softly bent. Hold a strap in one hand with your palm facing behind you and reach your opposite hand behind you to grasp the other end of the strap.

2. Inhale, keep your back straight, and roll your shoulders back and down.

3. Exhale and fold yourself forward, hinging at your hips to draw your torso toward your thighs and the top of your head toward floor. Allow your arms to move forward while you continue to hold the strap. Hold this stretch.

CHANGE IT UP

- For an easier version of this stretch and more support, ditch the strap and use a chair. Perform this stretch as described while facing the seat of a sturdy chair, resting your elbows and forearms on the chair seat for support. Focus on stretching your hamstrings and back within a range of motion that is comfortable for you.

- To deepen the stretch, skip the strap, interlace your fingers, and draw your knuckles toward the ceiling.

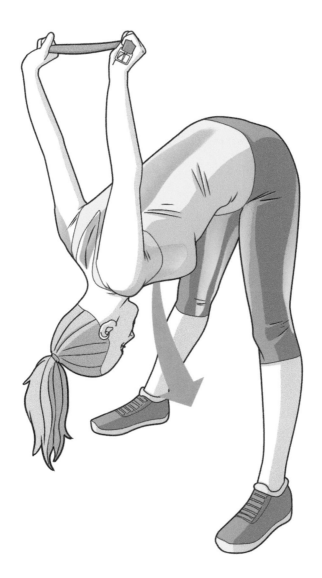

Allow the top of your head to move toward the floor during this forward fold to reduce tension in the back.

ASSISTED LOW LUNGE

Thighs (*quadriceps*) and hips (*hip flexors*)

This stretch targets your quads and hip flexors, muscles that are often strong but tight. If you spend long periods of time seated at work or run or cycle often, include this stretch in your flexibility training.

COOL DOWN • STATIC • PROP (TOWEL OR PILLOW)

INSTRUCTIONS

1. Start by kneeling on a folded towel or thin pillow with your toes tucked under and the balls of your feet pressed against a wall. Step your right foot forward, bending your right knee about 90 degrees. Keep your right knee in line with the second toe of your right foot.

2. Slide your left knee back slightly so the top of your foot is now resting against the wall and your toes point toward the ceiling, creating a stretch on the top of your left thigh and in your hip. Hold this stretch with your hands on top of your thigh.

3. Switch sides and repeat.

CHANGE IT UP

- For a little variety, use a strap to bend your left knee and draw your heel toward your glutes.

- To deepen the stretch in your hips and quads, lift your chest slightly while shifting your hips forward.

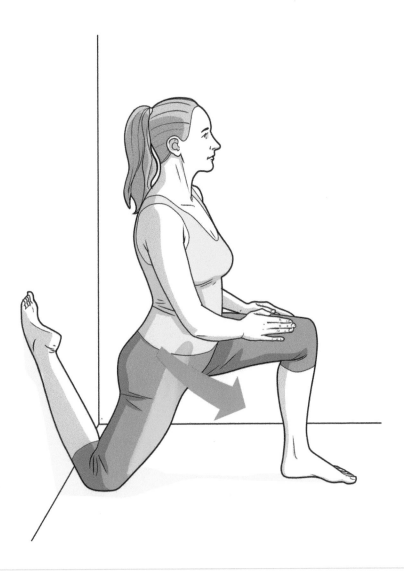

To reduce the risk of straining your front knee, keep that knee in line with the second toe of your front foot. This means you should be able to see the big toe of your front foot when doing this stretch. You can also choose to keep the toes of your back foot tucked as opposed to resting the top of your foot against the wall.

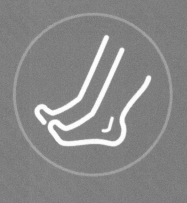

CHAPTER NINE

LOWER LEGS, ANKLES, and FEET

ANKLE CIRCLES

Lower legs/ankles

This dynamic range-of-motion exercise loosens your ankle joints, which can make you more comfortable when walking, running, and hiking. Additionally, making sure your ankle joints are able to move more freely can help reduce knee pain.

WARM UP • DYNAMIC

INSTRUCTIONS

1. Sit near the edge of a chair with both feet firmly planted on the floor and your hands resting on your thighs.

2. Lift your right foot off the floor and extend your right leg slightly away from your body.

3. Without moving your lifted leg, move your foot in a circular motion clockwise at the ankle. Complete this movement, then repeat it going counterclockwise.

4. Repeat with the left foot.

CHANGE IT UP

- If you need more support while keeping your leg up, lightly hold the back of your right thigh with both hands.

- To challenge yourself and test your balance, perform this exercise in a standing position with your hands on your hips.

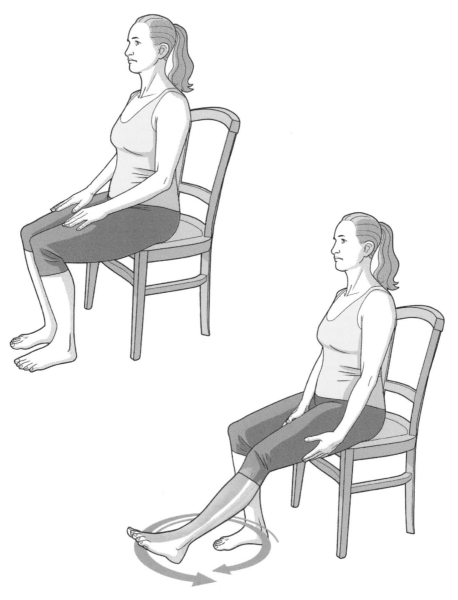

When moving your foot in circles at the ankle, really focus on each part of the movement: Move your ankle inward (turning the pinky-toe side of your foot slightly up), then point your toes down toward the ground, followed by moving your ankle outward (turning the big-toe side of your foot slightly up), and then point your toes up and pull them back toward your shin.

STANDING CALF STRETCH

Lower leg, ankles (*gastrocnemius and soleus*)

If you walk and climb stairs a lot or often wear high heels, which tighten your calf muscles, this stretch is key as it helps relieve pain in the both your ankles and knees.

COOL DOWN • STATIC

INSTRUCTIONS

1. Start in a split-stance position, facing a wall, with your left foot staggered in front of your right foot, shoulder-width apart. Place both hands on the wall for support. Your left foot, which is in front, should be 1 to 2 feet away from the wall, with your right foot 2 to 3 feet away from the wall.

2. With both heels pressed firmly into the floor, bend your left knee slightly while drawing your chest closer to the wall, creating a stretch in the back lower portion of your right leg. If you can, bend your elbows and place your palms and forearms flat against the wall, parallel to each other. Hold this stretch, then bring your right foot forward and put your left foot back.

3. Repeat.

CHANGE IT UP

- For a less intense stretch, lean your body only slightly forward, keeping only your palms planted on the wall and your chest farther away from it.

- To modify this stretch, instead of stepping your right foot back, place the toes of your right foot pointed up against the wall, with the ball of your foot parallel to floor and your heel firmly planted on the ground. Draw your chest closer to the wall to create the stretch in the back portion of the lower part of your right leg, as well as your right foot and toes.

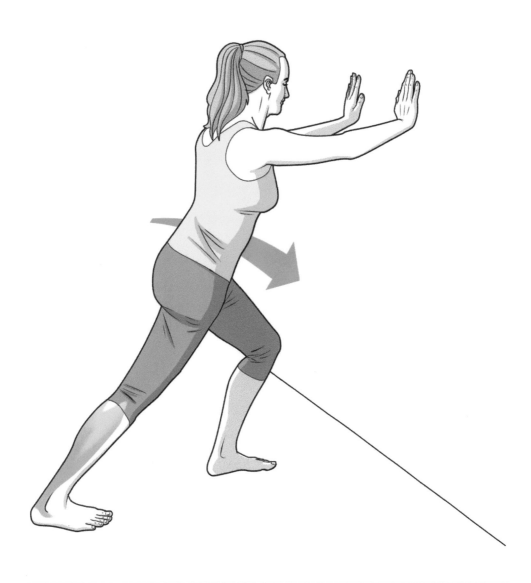

To get a good stretch in your calves, keep your back heel planted throughout the stretch and allow your front knee to bend slightly as you move your chest closer to the wall.

TIBIALIS ANTERIOR STRETCH

Lower leg/ankles (*tibialis anterior*)

This stretch relies on your body weight to target the muscles that run down the front side of your lower leg, such as the tibialis anterior, which can relieve some pain if you tend to get shin splints from walking, running, or hiking. Use a folded towel or do this stretch on a carpeted surface for more comfort and support.

COOL DOWN • STATIC • PROP (WALL OR CHAIR, TOWEL)

INSTRUCTIONS

1. With your feet together, stand parallel to a wall or chair and use your left hand for support.

2. Bend your right knee, draw your heel back, and place the top of your right foot on the floor, toes tucked under.

3. Keeping the top of your right foot in contact with the floor, shift your weight slightly forward to create a stretch in the front lower part of your leg. Hold this stretch for 3 to 5 breaths.

4. Switch sides and repeat with your left leg.

CHANGE IT UP

• If you need more support, do this stretch sitting at the edge of a chair and draw one foot slightly underneath the seat to place the top of that foot on the floor.

• To vary this stretch, explore different angles with your foot, positioning your heel slightly inward or outward, to change the focus of the stretch.

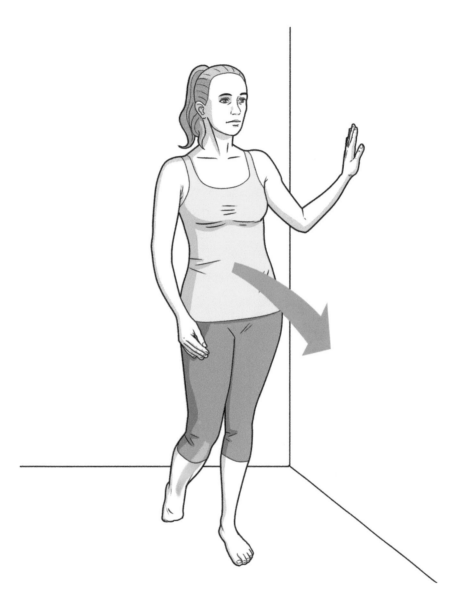

During this stretch, shift your weight forward as opposed to dragging your foot across the floor to reach your desired level of stretch.

SELF-MYOFASCIAL RELEASE FOR CALVES

Lower legs (*gastrocnemius and soleus*)

This technique targets the fascia (page 22) and calf muscles and improves the range of motion of your ankles, reducing your risk of ankle sprains. By placing your hands behind your body with your fingers pointed back, you'll stretch chest, shoulder, and arm muscles that can become tight as a result of poor posture. This exercise uses a foam roller.

WARM UP • COOL DOWN • PROP (FOAM ROLLER)

INSTRUCTIONS

1. Sit on the floor with both knees bent, feet flat on the floor. Plant both palms behind your body with your fingers angled away from your feet.

2. Keep your left knee bent and extend your right leg on top of a foam roller with your toes pointed up, positioning the roller underneath the back of your lower right leg.

3. Move your body back and forth on the foam roller at various angles, using small (2- to 6-inch) continuous movements, while applying gentle pressure to any tender areas.

4. Switch sides and repeat.

CHANGE IT UP

- To lessen any discomfort, apply pressure near, but not directly over, particularly tender areas and hold for up to 60 seconds. You may also want to angle your fingers slightly forward if your wrists bother you while doing this stretch.

- For an alternate position and more sensation, cross one leg over the other and position the foam roller directly over the tender area, applying pressure and holding the position for up to 30 seconds.

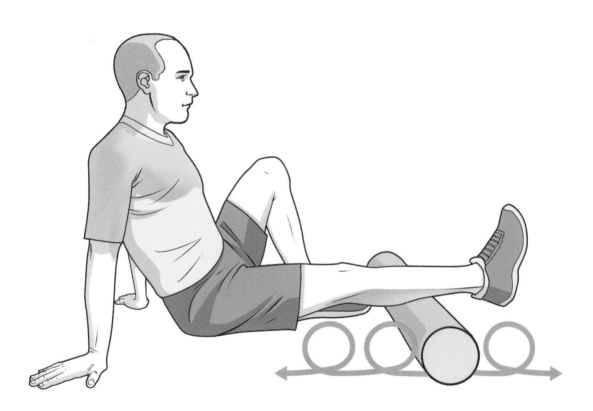

You can control the deepness of this stretch by applying more or less pressure, depending on your tolerance for discomfort. Be sure to breathe slowly and deeply through your nose to make this stretch even more relaxing. To get the most out of this move for your calf muscles, try different angles when rolling and keep your toes pointed up and toward your shin.

DOWNWARD-FACING DOG

Lower legs/ankles (*calves*), thighs (*hamstrings*), and back (*latissimus dorsi*)

One of the best-known yoga poses, this move stretches your hamstrings and calves while simultaneously strengthening your hands and arms.

COOL DOWN • STATIC

INSTRUCTIONS

1. Begin on your hands and knees, with your knees aligned below your hips and your hands slightly in front of your shoulders, fingers spread wide.

2. Press your palms firmly into the floor. Inhale while tucking your toes under.

3. Exhale while you extend your legs, lifting your hips and tailbone toward the ceiling to create an inverted *V* shape with your body, drawing the heels toward the floor while you maintain length in your spine. Hold this stretch.

CHANGE IT UP

- If this stretch seems too difficult, keep your knees bent to maintain length in your spine and place your hands on a pair of foam blocks.

- For a deeper stretch, raise yourself high onto the balls of your feet, then slowly lower your heels, pressing your feet firmly into the floor.

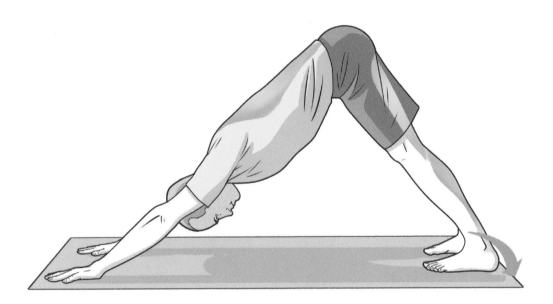

To ensure proper form for this yoga-inspired pose, engage your upper arms and allow your head and neck to remain positioned between your biceps as you hold this stretch. A strap can always be looped around your upper arms just above your elbows to remind you to keep your upper arms in.

PART THREE

The WORKOUTS

CHAPTER TEN

EVERYDAY ACTIVITIES

Workday Stretches

After you've spent hours working at a desk and typing on a computer, complete this workout to relieve the tightness in your chest, shoulders, neck, wrists, and hips.

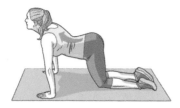

1.   Cat-Cow (8 repetitions) *page 70*

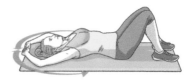

2.   Floor Angels (10 repetitions) *page 42*

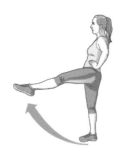

3.   Leg Swings (10 repetitions per side) *page 96*

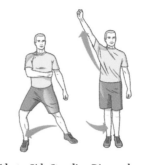

4.   Side-to-Side Standing Diagonals
     (8 repetitions per side) *page 100*

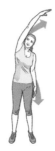

5.   Standing Crescent Moon (30 seconds per side)
     page 74

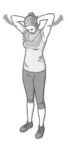

6.   Open-Heart Stretch (30 seconds) *page 44*

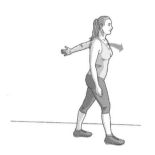

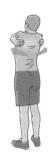

7. Biceps Stretch (30 seconds per side) *page 56*

8. Bear Hug (30 seconds) *page 76*

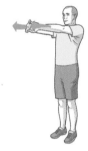

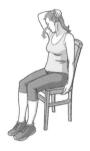

9. Wrist-Flexor Stretch (30 seconds) *page 62*

10. Seated Neck Stretch (30 seconds per side) *page 46*

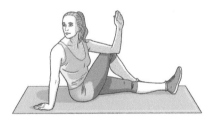

11. Half Lord of the Fishes (30 seconds per side) *page 88*

Stretches like Cat-Cow and Floor Angels can be modified to do in a seated position rather than on the floor (see "Change it Up" for each stretch), making this routine easy to do even while at the office.

Traveling Stretches

No matter where your journey takes you, complete this series of stretches to relieve the common aches and pains that set in after long hours of commuting or traveling.

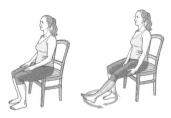

1. Ankle Circles (10 repetitions per side, 5 in each direction) *page 114*

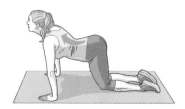

2. Cat-Cow (8 repetitions) *page 70*

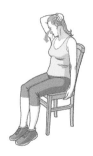

3. Seated Neck Stretch (30 seconds per side) *page 46*

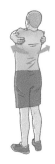

4. Bear Hug (30 seconds) *page 76*

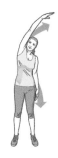

5. Standing Crescent Moon (30 seconds per side) *page 74*

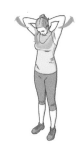

6. Open-Heart Stretch (30 seconds) *page 44*

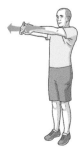

7. Wrist-Flexor Stretch (30 seconds) *page 62*

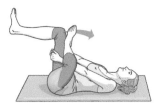

8. Figure 4 (30 seconds per side) *page 92*

Each stretch in this routine can be can be done in a seated position (see "Change It Up" for each stretch), so you can do this anywhere—whether on the road (although not while driving!) or in the air.

Morning Routine

Rise and shine with this dynamic stretching routine that will gradually get your blood flowing and awaken your body after a restful night's sleep. You'll be energized and ready for whatever the day may bring.

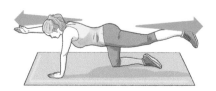

1. Floor Angels (10 repetitions) *page 42*

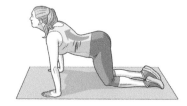

2. Cat-Cow (8 repetitions) *page 70*

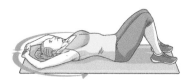

3. Bird-Dog (6 repetitions per side) *page 82*

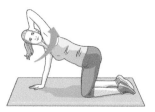

4. Quadruped Rotations (6 repetitions per side) *page 84*

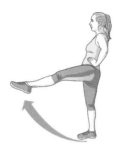

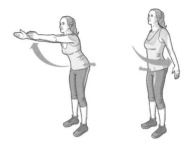

5. Leg Swings (10 repetitions per side) *page 96*

6. Hinge and Reach (10 repetitions) *page 50*

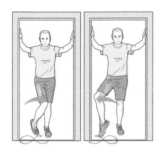

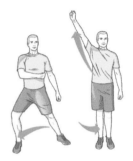

7. Figure 8 (8 repetitions per side) *page 98*

8. Side-to-Side Standing Diagonals (8 repetitions per side) *page 100*

You may find certain areas of your body feel particularly tight and stiff when you get up in the morning. Remember to listen to your body and work within a range of motion that feels comfortable for you.

Bedtime Routine

Static stretching is an ideal way to unwind and relieve some stress after a long day. This routine gives both your mind and body a chance to relax so you can enjoy a restful and rejuvenating night's sleep.

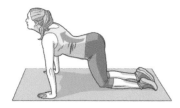

1. Cat-Cow (8 repetitions) *page 70*

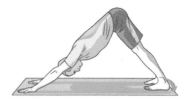

2. Downward-Facing Dog (30 seconds) *page 122*

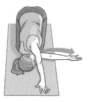

3. Thread the Needle (30 seconds per side) *page 40*

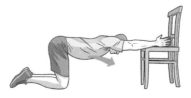

4. Kneeling Lat Stretch (30 seconds) *page 78*

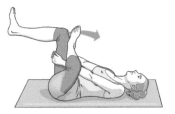

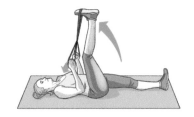

5. **Figure 4 (30 seconds per side)** *page 92*

6. **Assisted Supine Hamstring Stretch (30 seconds per side)** *page 104*

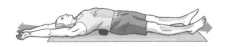

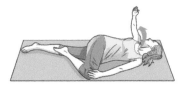

7. **Head-to-Toe Stretch (30 seconds)** *page 80*

8. **Supine Spinal Twist (30 seconds per side)** *page 72*

Muscles are best stretched when they are warm, so create an evening ritual for yourself by first enjoying a relaxing hot bath or shower before you begin these stretches.

While Watching TV

This easy-to-follow routine can be performed in your bedroom or living room while watching your favorite shows and movies. To maximize the effectiveness of these stretches, walk in place for the first 2 to 3 minutes to get the blood flowing and warm your muscles. You will need a foam roller for part of this routine.

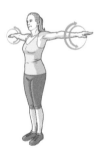

1. Self-Myofascial Release for Glutes
(30 seconds per side) *page 94*

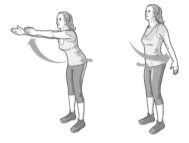

2. Hinge and Reach (10 repetitions) *page 50*

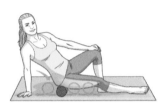

3. Arm Circles (10 repetitions per side,
5 in each direction) *page 48*

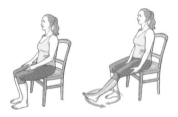

4. Ankle Circles (10 repetitions per side,
5 in each direction) *page 114*

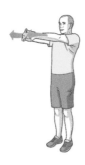

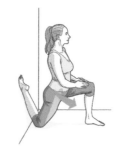

5. Wrist-Flexor Stretch (30 seconds) *page 62*

6. Assisted Low Lunge (30 seconds per side) *page 110*

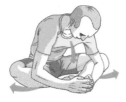

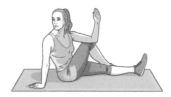

7. Bound Angle (30 seconds) *page 90*

8. Half Lord of the Fishes (30 seconds per side) *page 88*

When doing a stretch like the Half Lord of the Fishes, position yourself so your bent leg is always closest to the TV. This way, when you twist, you are turning toward the TV—you won't miss a minute of your favorite show!

After a Long Phone Call

After you've spent a while on the phone, use this series of stretches to loosen your neck, arms, forearms, and wrists, which often tighten up after holding the telephone in the same position for an extended period of time.

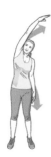

1. Arm Circles (10 repetitions per side, 5 in each direction) *page 48*

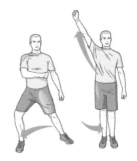

2. Side-to-Side Standing Diagonals (6 repetitions per side) *page 100*

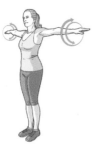

3. Standing Crescent Moon (30 seconds per side) *page 74*

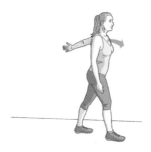

4. Biceps Stretch (30 seconds per side) *page 56*

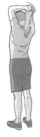

5. Overhead Triceps Stretch (30 seconds per side) *page 58*

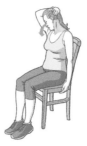

6. Seated Neck Stretch (30 seconds per side) *page 46*

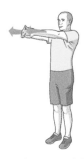

7. **Wrist-Flexor Stretch (30 seconds)** *page 62*

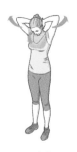

8. **Open-Heart Stretch (30 seconds)** *page 44*

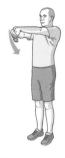

9. **Wrist-Extensor Stretch (30 seconds per side)** *page 60*

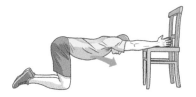

10. **Kneeling Lat Stretch (30 seconds)** *page 78*

If you're stuck on the phone, pace quietly back and forth, if possible, as a bit of a warm-up. You'll increase your muscle temperature, which makes these stretches even more effective once you've finished your call.

Gardening

Before you start digging in the dirt, prepare your body with this combination of dynamic and static stretches that target your back and hips and will lessen any tightness and stiffness you might feel following weeding and planting.

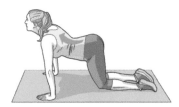

1. Cat-Cow (8 repetitions) *page 70*

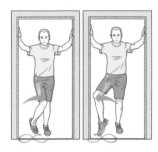

2. Bird-Dog (6 repetitions per side) *page 82*

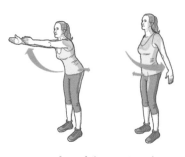

3. Hinge and Reach (10 repetitions) *page 50*

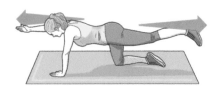

4. Figure 8 (8 repetitions per side) *page 98*

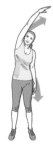

5. Standing Crescent Moon (30 seconds per side) *page 74*

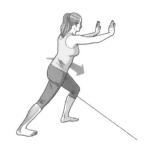

6. Standing Calf Stretch (30 seconds per side) *page 116*

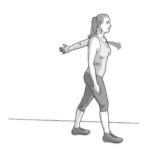

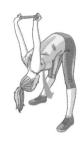

7. Biceps Stretch (30 seconds per side) *page 56*

8. Wide-Legged Forward Fold with Chest Expansion (30 seconds) *page 108*

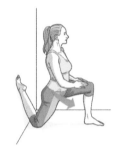

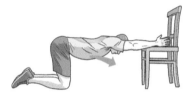

9. Assisted Low Lunge (30 seconds per side) *page 110*

10. Kneeling Lat Stretch (30 seconds) *page 78*

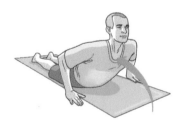

11. Low Cobra (30 seconds) *page 68*

In addition to following this stretching routine, be sure to use good posture and body mechanics, such as hinging at the hips, a movement pattern the Hinge and Reach stretch helps, to lessen any tension and discomfort you may feel while working in the yard.

Shoveling Snow

If snow is a regular winter occurrence in your area, complete this series of stretches before heading out to clear your driveway or sidewalk so your muscles are prepared for the heavy lifting and repeated twisting needed for shoveling. You will need a foam roller for part of this sequence.

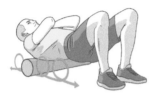

1. Self-Myofascial Release for Mid and Upper Back (60 seconds) *page 66*

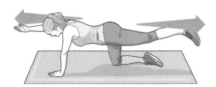

2. Bird-Dog (6 repetitions per side) *page 82*

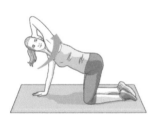

3. Quadruped Rotations (6 repetitions per side) *page 84*

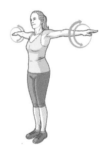

4. Arm Circles (10 repetitions per side, 5 in each direction) *page 48*

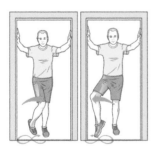

5. Figure 8 (8 repetitions per side) *page 98*

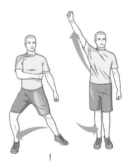

6. Side-to-Side Standing Diagonals (6 repetitions per side) *page 100*

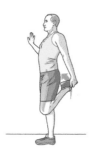

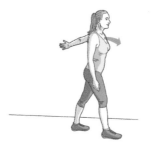

7. Supported Standing Quadriceps Stretch (30 seconds per side) *page 106*

8. Biceps Stretch (30 seconds per side) *page 56*

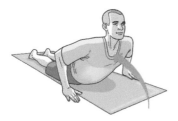

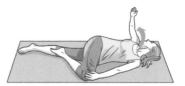

9. Low Cobra (30 seconds per side) *page 68*

10. Supine Spinal Twist (30 seconds per side) *page 72*

To protect the lower back, Self-Myofascial Release for Mid and Upper Back is a key move in this series. It increases the range of motion in your thoracic spine, a key series of joints used to rotate your upper body, a basic movement when shoveling snow.

Heavy Lifting

Whether you're cleaning out the garage, moving into a new house, or carrying boxes at work, this routine includes dynamic stretches for your hips and back to help you stay safe and move with ease.

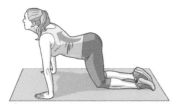

1. Cat-Cow (8 repetitions) *page 70*

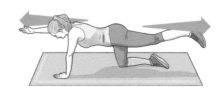

2. Bird-Dog (6 repetitions per side) *page 82*

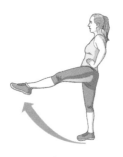

3. Leg Swings (10 repetitions per side) *page 96*

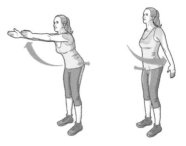

4. Hinge and Reach (10 repetitions) *page 50*

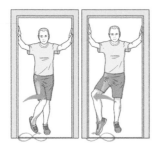

5. Figure 8 (8 repetitions per side) *page 98*

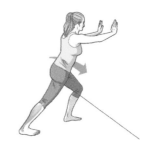

6. Standing Calf Stretch (30 seconds per side) *page 116*

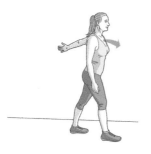

7. Biceps Stretch (30 seconds per side) *page 56*

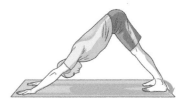

8. Downward-Facing Dog (30 seconds) *page 122*

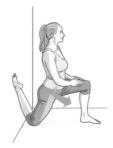

9. Assisted Low Lunge (30 seconds per side) *page 110*

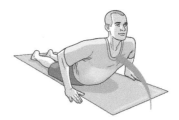

10. Low Cobra (30 seconds) *page 68*

I include static stretches in this routine to target your biceps, which can become tight after hauling heavy weight in a bent-arm (flexed) position.

CHAPTER ELEVEN

ACTIVE LIVING

Walking

Since walking is a regular part of our daily lives as well as many people's main form of physical activity, I specifically designed this before-and-after series of stretches to help you walk with greater ease.

BEFORE

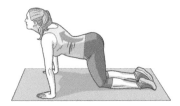

1.   Cat-Cow (8 repetitions) *page 70*

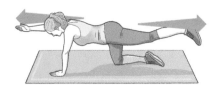

2.   Bird-Dog (6 repetitions per side) *page 82*

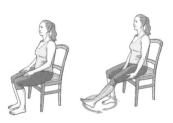

3.   Ankle Circles (10 repetitions per side, 5 in each direction) *page 114*

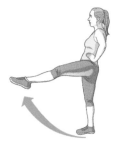

4.   Leg Swings (10 repetitions per side) *page 96*

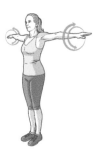

5.   Arm Circles (10 repetitions per side, 5 in each direction) *page 48*

AFTER

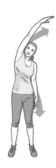

1. Standing Crescent Moon (30 seconds per side)
    page 74

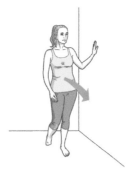

2. Tibialis Anterior Stretch (30 seconds per side)
    page 118

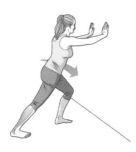

3. Standing Calf Stretch (30 seconds
    per side) *page 116*

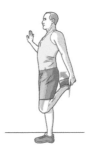

4. Supported Standing Quadriceps Stretch
    (30 seconds per side) *page 106*

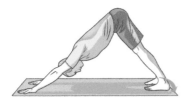

5. Downward-Facing Dog (30 seconds) *page 122*

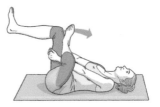

6. Figure 4 (30 seconds per side) *page 92*

According to the American College of Sports Medicine, static stretching is most effective when the muscles are warm, so the "After" sequence is perfect following a nice stroll.

Running

To keep you up and running and pain-free, I put together this series of before-and-after stretches to focus on the muscles of your lower leg, namely the tibialis anterior, gastrocnemius, and soleus. Following this routine will reduce the likelihood of getting shin splints or suffering ankle sprains. You will need a foam roller for part of this sequence.

BEFORE

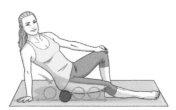

1. Self-Myofascial Release for Glutes
(30 seconds per side) *page 94*

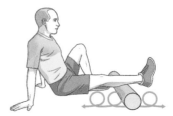

2. Self-Myofascial Release for Calves
(30 seconds per side) *page 120*

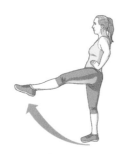

3. Leg Swings (10 repetitions per side) *page 96*

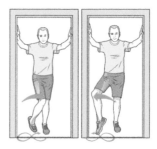

4. Figure 8 (8 repetitions per side) *page 98*

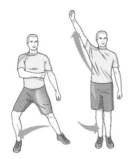

5. Side-to-Side Standing Diagonals
(6 repetitions per side) *page 100*

AFTER

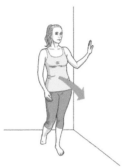

1. Tibialis Anterior Stretch (30 seconds per side)
    page 118

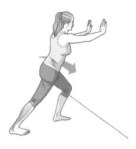

2. Standing Calf Stretch (30 seconds per side) *page 116*

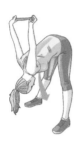

3. Wide-Legged Forward Fold with Chest Expansion (30 seconds) *page 108*

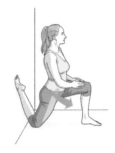

4. Assisted Low Lunge (30 seconds per side)
    page 110

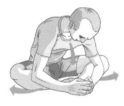

5. Bound Angle (30 seconds) *page 90*

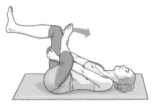

6. Figure 4 (30 seconds per side) *page 92*

Being that the calf muscles (gastrocnemius and soleus) are attached to your Achilles tendon, regularly stretching these muscles helps prevent tendinitis of the Achilles tendon, a chronic inflammation that makes walking and running painful.

Swimming

Swimming is a low-impact, full-body workout. This before-and-after series stretches the body from head to toe, with specific focus on your back and shoulders so you can improve your stroke while avoiding any shoulder pain or discomfort. You will need a foam roller for part of this sequence.

BEFORE

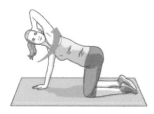

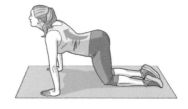

1. Self-Myofascial Release for Mid and Upper Back (60 seconds) *page 66*

2. Floor Angels (8 repetitions) *page 42*

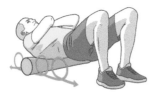

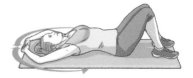

3. Quadruped Rotations (6 repetitions per side) *page 84*

4. Cat-Cow (8 repetitions) *page 70*

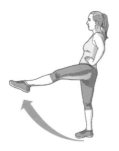

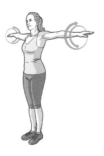

5. Leg Swings (10 repetitions per side) *page 96*

6. Arm Circles (10 repetitions per side, 5 in each direction) *page 48*

AFTER

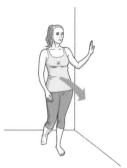

1. Tibialis Anterior Stretch (30 seconds per side)
page 118

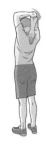

2. Overhead Triceps Stretch (30 seconds per side) *page 58*

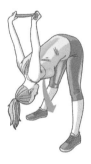

3. Wide-Legged Forward Fold with Chest Expansion (30 seconds) *page 108*

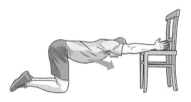

4. Kneeling Lat Stretch (30 seconds) *page 78*

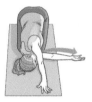

5. Thread the Needle (30 seconds per side) *page 40*

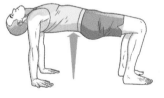

6. Reverse Tabletop (30 seconds) *page 52*

Stretching the latissimus dorsi, the large muscle of the back, can help reduce your risk of suffering a rotator cuff injury.

Cycling

After a long bike ride on the open road, your hips, chest, and abdominals can become tight from being in a flexed position. I created these before-and-after stretch sequences to warm and loosen these muscle groups. You will need a foam roller for part of this sequence.

BEFORE

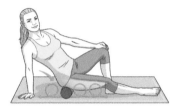

1. Self-Myofascial Release for Glutes
    (30 seconds per side) *page 94*

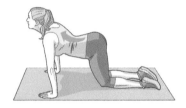

2. Cat-Cow (8 repetitions) *page 70*

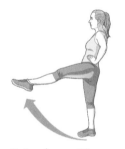

3. Leg Swings (10 repetitions per side) *page 96*

AFTER

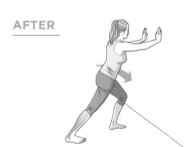

1. Standing Calf Stretch (30 seconds
    per side) *page 116*

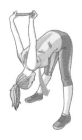

2. Wide-Legged Forward Fold with Chest
    Expansion (30 seconds) *page 108*

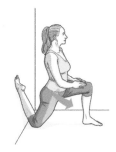

3. Assisted Low Lunge (30 seconds per side) *page 110*

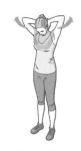

4. Open-Heart Stretch (30 seconds) *page 44*

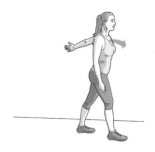

5. Biceps Stretch (30 seconds per side) *page 56*

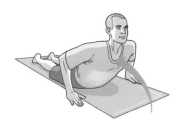

6. Low Cobra (30 seconds) *page 68*

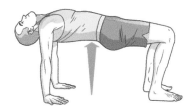

7. Reverse Tabletop (30 seconds) *page 52*

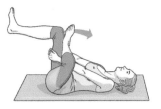

8. Figure 4 (30 seconds per side) *page 92*

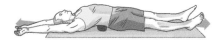

9. Head-to-Toe Stretch (30 seconds) *page 80*

Since your elbows are in a bent (flexed) position along with the rest of your body while cycling, the Biceps Stretch in this routine is intended to help prevent pain in your elbows.

Golf

This routine starts with dynamic stretches to warm you before you hit the links and is designed to increase mobility in the upper back. Loosening this area of your body allows you to produce the rotational movements needed for the perfect golf stroke—and score. You will need a foam roller for part of this sequence.

BEFORE

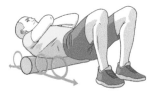

1. Self-Myofascial Release for Mid and Upper Back (30 seconds per side) *page 66*

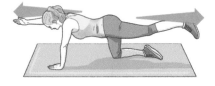

2. Bird-Dog (6 repetitions per side) *page 82*

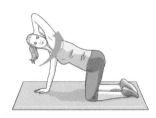

3. Quadruped Rotations (6 repetitions per side) *page 84*

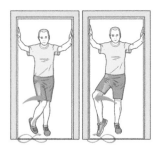

4. Figure 8 (8 repetitions per side) *page 98*

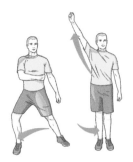

5. Side-to-Side Standing Diagonals (6 repetitions per side) *page 100*

AFTER

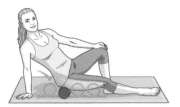

1. Self-Myofascial Release for Glutes (30 seconds per side) *page 94*

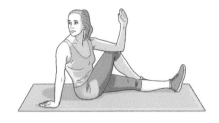

2. Half Lord of the Fishes (30 seconds per side) *page 88*

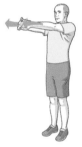

3. Wrist-Flexor Stretch (30 seconds) *page 62*

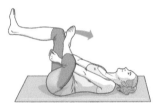

4. Figure 4 (30 seconds per side) *page 92*

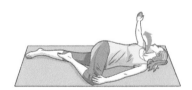

5. Supine Spinal Twist (30 seconds per side) *page 72*

I incorporate the Half Lord of the Fishes in this sequence to offset any muscle imbalances you might have as a result of repetitive movements in one direction, such as from your golf swing.

Dancing

Dancing is a fun and dynamic form of physical activity that includes a full range of movements. Appropriately, this series of before-and-after stretches prepares your body to move smoothly and safely (and gracefully) in any given direction.

BEFORE

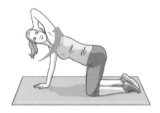

1. Cat-Cow (8 repetitions) *page 70*

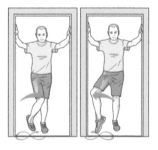

2. Quadruped Rotations (6 repetitions per side) *page 84*

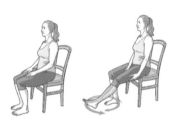

3. Ankle Circles (10 repetitions per side, 5 in each direction) *page 114*

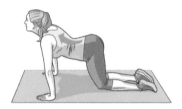

4. Figure 8 (6 repetitions per side) *page 98*

AFTER

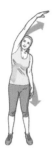

1. Standing Crescent Moon (30 seconds per side)
    page 74

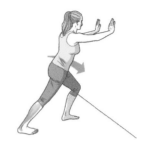

2. Standing Calf Stretch (30 seconds per side) *page 116*

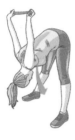

3. Wide-Legged Forward Fold with Chest Expansion (30 seconds) *page 108*

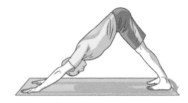

4. Downward-Facing Dog (30 seconds) *page 122*

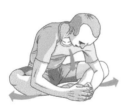

5. Bound Angle (30 seconds) *page 90*

Improve your ankle mobility with stretches such as Ankle Circles, Standing Calf Stretch, and Downward-Facing Dog to lessen your risk of ankle sprains.

Tennis

Whether you enjoy a leisurely or competitive game of tennis, I include here both dynamic and static moves for your hips to prepare you for the quick changes in speed and direction this potentially fast-paced sport is known for. You will need a foam roller for part of this sequence.

BEFORE

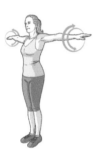

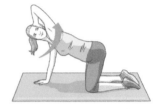

1.   Self-Myofascial Release for Mid and Upper Back (60 seconds) *page 66*

2.   Quadruped Rotations (6 repetitions per side) *page 84*

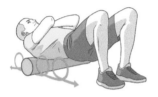

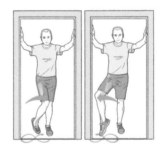

3.   Arm Circles (10 repetitions per side, 5 in each direction) *page 48*

4.   Figure 8 (6 repetitions per side) *page 98*

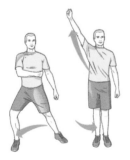

5.   Side-to-Side Standing Diagonals (8 repetitions per side) *page 100*

AFTER

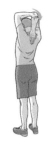

1. Overhead Triceps Stretch (30 seconds per side) *page 58*

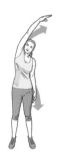

2. Standing Crescent Moon (30 seconds per side) *page 74*

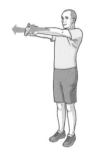

3. Wrist-Flexor Stretch (30 seconds per side) *page 62*

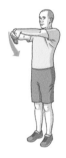

4. Wrist-Extensor Stretch (30 seconds per side) *page 60*

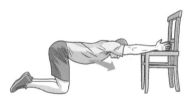

5. Kneeling Lat Stretch (30 seconds) *page 78*

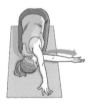

6. Thread the Needle (30 seconds per side) *page 40*

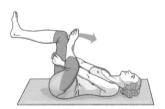

7. Figure 4 (30 seconds per side) *page 92*

Given the nature of a racket sport like tennis, it's important to perform stretches for the forearm muscles, which both flex and extend the wrists.

Hiking

Given that we use our legs so much when going up and down hills during a hike, I created a sequence of before-and-after stretches that focuses on stretching the major muscles of the lower body, included the hamstrings, glutes, and calves. You will need a foam roller for part of this sequence.

BEFORE

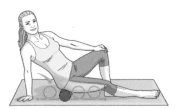

1. Self-Myofascial Release for Glutes (30 seconds per side) *page 94*

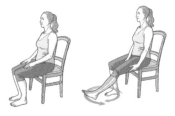

2. Ankle Circles (10 repetitions per side, 5 in each direction) *page 114*

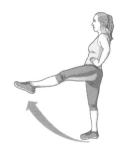

3. Leg Swings (10 repetitions per side) *page 96*

AFTER

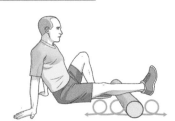

1. Self-Myofascial Release for Calves (30 seconds per side) *page 120*

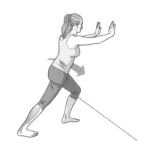

2. Standing Calf Stretch (30 seconds per side) *page 116*

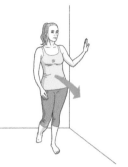

3. Tibialis Anterior Stretch (30 seconds per side)
page 118

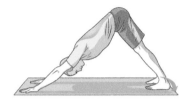

4. Downward-Facing Dog (30 seconds) *page 122*

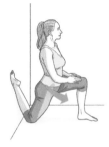

5. Assisted Low Lunge (30 seconds per side)
page 110

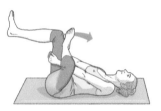

6. Figure 4 (30 seconds per side) *page 92*

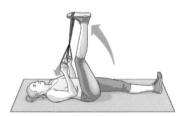

7. Assisted Supine Hamstring Stretch
(30 seconds per side) *page 104*

When you stretch your lower-leg muscles, such as the tibialis anterior, you lessen your risk for developing shin splints.

Baseball/Softball

With all the throwing, swinging, and reaching involved in playing baseball and softball, you'll want to keep your upper back and shoulders loose. I've built dynamic and static stretches for your shoulders into this before-and-after sequence to help you improve some key skills, such as throwing. You will need a foam roller for part of this sequence.

BEFORE

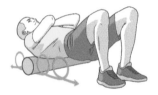

1. Self-Myofascial Release for Mid and Upper Back (60 seconds) *page 66*

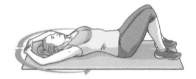

2. Floor Angels (10 repetitions) *page 42*

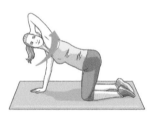

3. Quadruped Rotations (6 repetitions per side) *page 84*

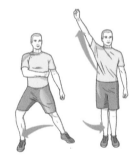

4. Side-to-Side Standing Diagonals (8 repetitions per side) *page 100*

AFTER

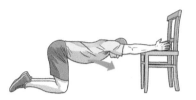

1.   Kneeling Lat Stretch (30 seconds) *page 78*

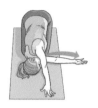

2.   Thread the Needle (30 seconds per side) *page 40*

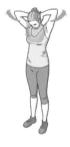

3.   Open-Heart Stretch (30 seconds) *page 44*

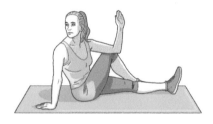

4.   Half Lord of the Fishes (30 seconds per side) *page 88*

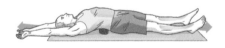

5.   Head-to-Toe Stretch (30 seconds) *page 80*

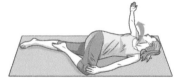

6.   Supine Spinal Twist (30 seconds per side) *page 72*

Thread the Needle is a great stretch for your shoulders if you suffer from bursitis or tendinitis, since it helps reduce the pain caused by these conditions.

Cross-Country Skiing

This series of before-and-after stretches includes some dynamic movements for your hips, which can become tight and stiff while you cross-country ski. You will need a foam roller for part of this sequence.

BEFORE

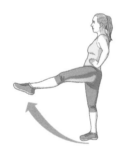

1. Self-Myofascial Release for Glutes (30 seconds per side) *page 94*

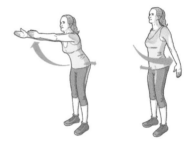

2. Hinge and Reach (10 repetitions) *page 50*

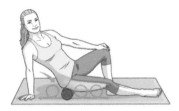

3. Leg Swings (10 repetitions per side) *page 96*

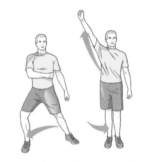

4. Side-to-Side Standing Diagonals (8 repetitions per side) *page 100*

AFTER

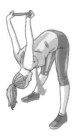

1. Wide-Legged Forward Fold with Chest Expansion (30 seconds) *page 108*

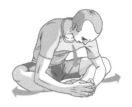

2. Bound Angle (30 seconds) *page 90*

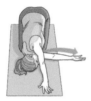

3. Thread the Needle (30 seconds per side) *page 40*

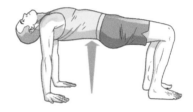

4. Reverse Tabletop (30 seconds) *page 52*

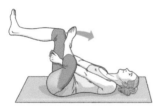

5. Figure 4 (30 seconds per side) *page 92*

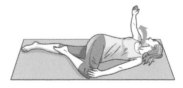

6. Supine Spinal Twist (30 seconds per side) *page 72*

Effectively stretching your inner thighs (the hip adductors) and outer thighs (the hip abductors) with moves like Bound Angle and Figure 4 can enhance stability in your knees.

Upper-Body Resistance Training

This before-and-after series of stretches focuses on the major muscles of your upper body—such as your chest and shoulders. You will need a foam roller for part of this sequence.

BEFORE

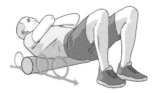

1. Self-Myofascial Release for Mid and Upper Back (60 seconds per side) *page 66*

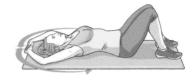

2. Floor Angels (8 repetitions) *page 42*

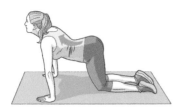

3. Cat-Cow (8 repetitions) *page 70*

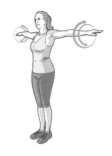

4. Arm Circles (10 repetitions per side, 5 in each direction) *page 48*

AFTER

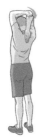

1. Overhead Triceps Stretch (30 seconds per side) *page 58*

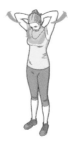

2. Open-Heart Stretch (30 seconds) *page 44*

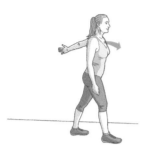

3. Biceps Stretch (30 seconds per side) *page 56*

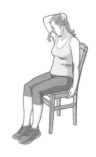

4. Seated Neck Stretch (30 seconds per side) *page 46*

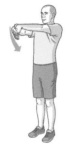

5. Wrist-Extensor Stretch (30 seconds per side) *page 60*

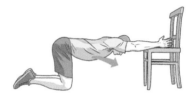

6. Kneeling Lat Stretch (30 seconds) *page 78*

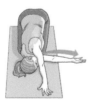

7. Thread the Needle (30 seconds per side) *page 40*

When you use a foam roller, allow your upper back to gently arch and drape over the roller. This movement, together with the back-and-forth rolling motion, loosens your shoulders and makes upper-body strength-training exercises, like shoulder presses, easier.

Upper-Body Resistance Training   169

Lower-Body Resistance Training

This before-and-after series of stretches focuses on the major muscles of your lower body, such as your glutes, hamstrings, and quadriceps, commonly worked during strength training. You will need a foam roller for part of this sequence.

BEFORE

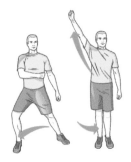

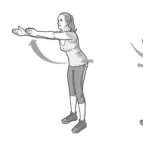

1.   Leg Swings (10 repetitions per side) *page 96*

2.   Hinge and Reach (10 repetitions) *page 50*

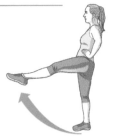

3.   Side-to-Side Standing Diagonals (8 repetitions per side) *page 100*

AFTER

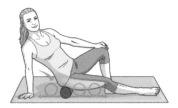

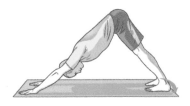

1.   Self-Myofascial Release for Glutes (30 seconds per side) *page 94*

2.   Downward-Facing Dog (30 seconds) *page 122*

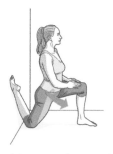

3. Assisted Low Lunge (30 seconds per side) *page 110*

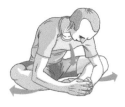

4. Bound Angle (30 seconds) *page 90*

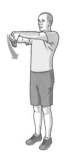

5. Wrist-Extensor Stretch (30 seconds per side) *page 60*

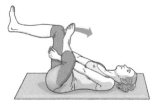

6. Figure 4 (30 seconds per side) *page 92*

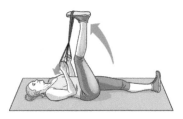

7. Assisted Supine Hamstring Stretch (30 seconds per side) *page 104*

Because you might do lower-body exercises, like squats and lunges, while holding dumbbells or a barbell, I include a Wrist-Extensor Stretch in this routine to stretch the forearm muscles.

CHAPTER TWELVE

EASING ACHES and PAINS

Stiff Neck

Effectively stretching your neck and upper back can help reduce pain and discomfort in these areas as well as potentially relieve headaches. You will need a foam roller for part of this sequence.

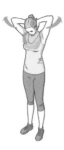

1. **Self-Myofascial Release for Mid and Upper Back (60 seconds)** *page 66*

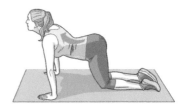

2. **Cat-Cow (8 repetitions)** *page 70*

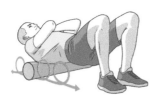

3. **Open-Heart Stretch (30 seconds)** *page 44*

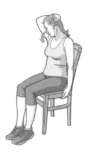

4. **Seated Neck Stretch (30 seconds per side)** *page 46*

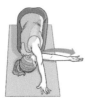

5. **Thread the Needle (30 seconds per side)** *page 40*

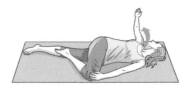

6. **Supine Spinal Twist (30 seconds per side)** *page 72*

Cat-Cow is more of a motion exercise than a stretch. Instead of holding the end of the move for a bit, which can strain your neck, perform this dynamic stretch fluidly using your inhalations and exhalations to set the tempo.

Sore Wrists and Elbows

To ease pain from tennis elbow, carpal tunnel syndrome, golfer's elbow, and the like, I include stretches for muscles that act on your elbow, as well as those that act on your wrists, including your biceps, triceps, and forearm muscles.

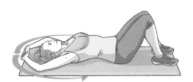

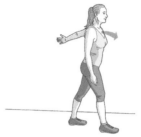

1.   Floor Angels (10 repetitions) *page 42*

2.   Biceps Stretch (30 seconds per side) *page 56*

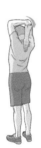

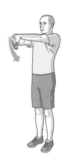

3.   Overhead Triceps Stretch (30 seconds per side) *page 58*

4.   Wrist-Extensor Stretch (30 seconds per side) *page 60*

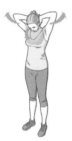

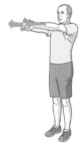

5.   Open-Heart Stretch (30 seconds) *page 44*

6.   Wrist-Flexor Stretch (30 seconds) *page 62*

The Wrist-Flexor and Wrist-Extensor stretches address tightness in your forearms and wrists, which may become tight after long periods of typing.

Frozen Shoulder

To relieve pain and stiffness in your shoulder joint, this series of stretches includes dynamic range-of-motion exercises. You will need a foam roller for part of this sequence.

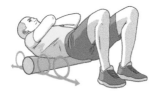

1. Self-Myofascial Release for Mid and Upper Back (60 seconds) *page 66*

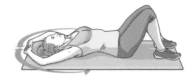

2. Floor Angels (10 repetitions) *page 42*

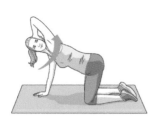

3. Quadruped Rotations (6 repetitions per side) *page 84*

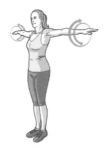

4. Arm Circles (10 repetitions per side, 5 in each direction) *page 48*

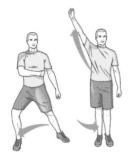

5. Side-to-Side Standing Diagonals (8 repetitions per side) *page 100*

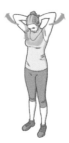

6. Open-Heart Stretch (30 seconds) *page 44*

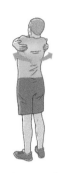

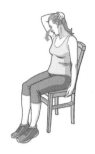

7. **Bear Hug (30 seconds)** *page 76*

8. **Seated Neck Stretch (30 seconds per side)** *page 46*

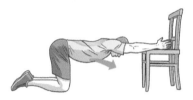

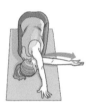

9. **Kneeling Lat Stretch (30 seconds)** *page 78*

10. **Thread the Needle (30 seconds per side)** *page 40*

In addition to dynamic stretches, static stretches like the Bear Hug can help minimize shoulder-related issues.

Tight Hips

This series of stretches is designed to alleviate the stiffness you get from sitting for prolonged periods of time. You will need a foam roller for part of this sequence.

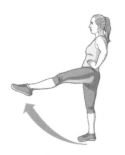

1.　Self-Myofascial Release for Glutes (30 seconds per side) *page 94*

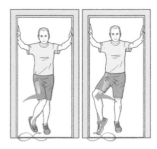

2.　Hinge and Reach (10 repetitions) *page 50*

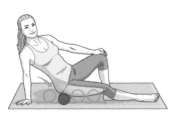

3.　Leg Swings (10 repetitions per side) *page 96*

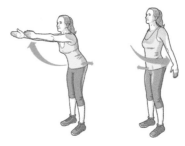

4.　Figure 8 (8 repetitions per side) *page 98*

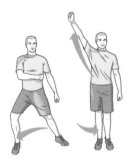

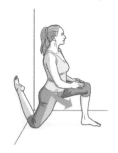

5. Side-to-Side Standing Diagonals
(8 repetitions per side) *page 100*

6. Assisted Low Lunge (30 seconds per side)
page 110

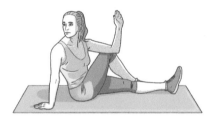

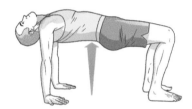

7. Half Lord of the Fishes (30 seconds per side)
page 88

8. Reverse Tabletop (30 seconds) *page 52*

Moves like the Reverse Tabletop can help stretch your hips while simultaneously strengthening your glutes (buttocks), which often become weakened when you have tightness in your hips.

Sore Knees and Ankles

To reduce discomfort in the quadriceps, hamstrings, and calves, this series of stretches focuses on the major muscles of your legs. You will need a foam roller for part of this sequence.

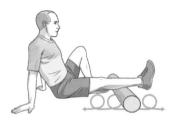

1. Self-Myofascial Release for Calves (30 seconds per side) *page 120*

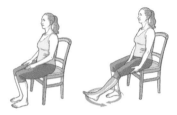

2. Ankle Circles (10 repetitions per side, 5 in each direction) *page 114*

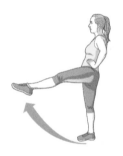

3. Leg Swings (10 repetitions per side) *page 96*

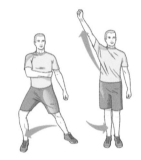

4. Side-to-Side Standing Diagonals (6 repetitions per side) *page 100*

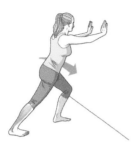

5. Standing Calf Stretch (30 seconds per side) *page 116*

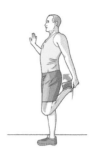

6. Supported Standing Quadriceps Stretch (30 seconds per side) *page 106*

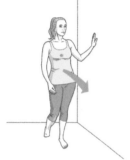

7. Tibialis Anterior Stretch (30 seconds per side) *page 118*

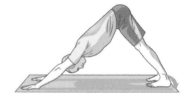

8. Downward-Facing Dog (30 seconds) *page 122*

Stretching the back of your lower leg can improve mobility in your ankle joint, which can relieve some pain in both your ankles and knees.

Arthritis

For individuals with arthritis, this series of dynamic stretches lubricates the joints, helping increase and maintain range of motion and making movements more comfortable.

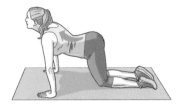

1. Cat-Cow (8 repetitions) *page 70*

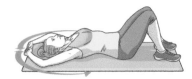

2. Floor Angels (8 repetitions) *page 42*

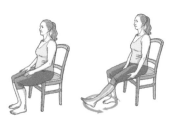

3. Ankle Circles (10 repetitions per side, 5 in each direction) *page 114*

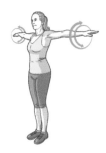

4. Arm Circles (10 repetitions per side, 5 in each direction) *page 48*

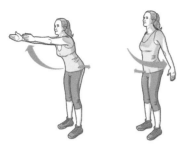

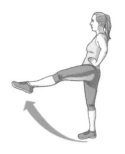

5. **Hinge and Reach (10 repetitions)** *page 50*

6. **Leg Swings (10 repetitions per side)** *page 96*

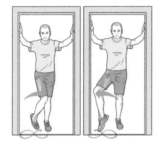

7. **Figure 8 (8 repetitions per side)** *page 98*

Start off slowly, and with a small range of motion, when doing each stretch so your body has ample time to warm up.

Diabetes

Stretching is not only beneficial for increasing flexibility. Several studies have found that static stretching may also help regulate blood glucose levels if you have diabetes.

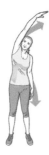

1. Standing Crescent Moon (30 seconds per side)
   page 74

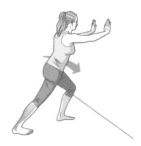

2. Standing Calf Stretch (30 seconds per side) *page 116*

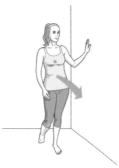

3. Tibialis Anterior Stretch (30 seconds per side)
   page 118

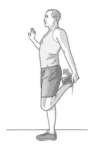

4. Supported Standing Quadriceps Stretch (30 seconds per side) *page 106*

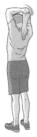

5. Overhead Triceps Stretch (30 seconds per side) *page 58*

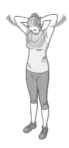

6. Open-Heart Stretch (30 seconds) *page 44*

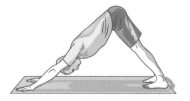

7. Downward-Facing Dog (30 seconds) *page 122*

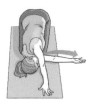

8. Thread the Needle (30 seconds per side) *page 40*

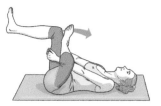

9. Figure 4 (30 seconds per side) *page 92*

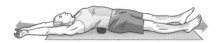

10. Head-to-Toe Stretch (30 seconds) *page 80*

For a more comfortable stretching experience, walk around the block or simply walk in place for several minutes before performing these static stretches to get your blood flowing and your muscles warmed up.

CHAPTER THIRTEEN

SPECIALIZED ROUTINES

General Warm-Up

This active warm-up will prepare you for just about any type of workout. The inclusion of self-myofascial release and dynamic range-of-motion stretches will increase your core body temperature and improve your mobility. You will need a foam roller for part of this sequence.

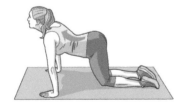

1. Self-Myofascial Release for Mid and Upper Back (60 seconds) *page 66*

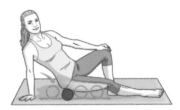

2. Self-Myofascial Release for Glutes (30 seconds per side) *page 94*

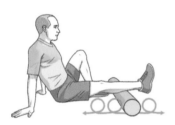

3. Self-Myofascial Release for Calves (30 seconds per side) *page 120*

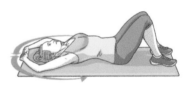

4. Floor Angels (8 repetitions) *page 42*

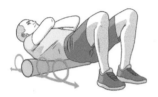

5. Cat-Cow (6 repetitions) *page 70*

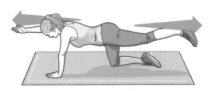

6. Bird-Dog (6 repetitions per side) *page 82*

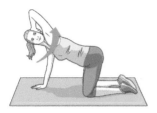

7. Quadruped Rotations (6 repetitions per side) *page 84*

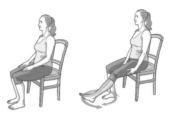

8. Ankle Circles (10 repetitions per side, 5 in each direction) *page 114*

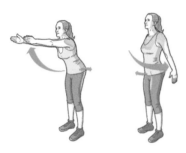

9. Hinge and Reach (8 repetitions) *page 50*

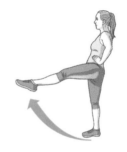

10. Leg Swings (8 repetitions per side) *page 96*

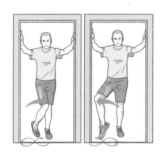

11. Figure 8 (8 repetitions per side) *page 98*

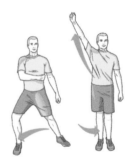

12. Side-to-Side Standing Diagonals (6 repetitions per side) *page 100*

By improving tissue density first through self-myofascial release, you can relieve tension, increase blood flow, improve mobility, and enhance your overall movement throughout your body.

General Cool-Down

Perfect for post-exercise, I've designed this series of stretches to loosen the major muscle groups typically used in daily activities, including your calves, thighs, hips, torso, back, chest, and shoulders.

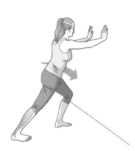

1. Standing Calf Stretch (30 seconds per side) *page 116*

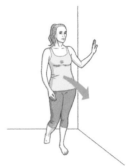

2. Tibialis Anterior Stretch (30 seconds per side) *page 118*

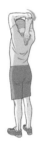

3. Overhead Triceps Stretch (30 seconds per side) *page 58*

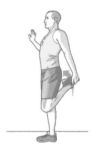

4. Supported Standing Quadriceps Stretch (30 seconds per side) *page 106*

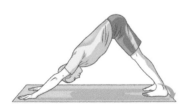

5. Downward-Facing Dog (30 seconds) *page 122*

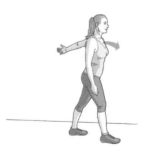

6. Biceps Stretch (30 seconds per side) *page 56*

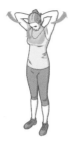

7. Open-Heart Stretch (30 seconds) *page 44*

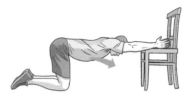

8. Kneeling Lat Stretch (30 seconds) *page 78*

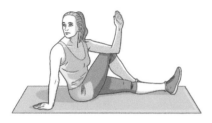

9. Half Lord of the Fishes (30 seconds per side) *page 88*

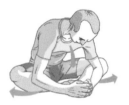

10. Bound Angle (30 seconds) *page 90*

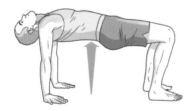

11. Reverse Tabletop (30 seconds) *page 52*

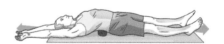

12. Head-to-Toe Stretch (30 seconds) *page 80*

If you have extra time, perform each of these static stretches twice, holding the stretch for 30 seconds, resting for 15 seconds, and repeating for 30 seconds, totaling 60 seconds per stretch.

Yoga-Inspired

As the name implies, I created this yoga-inspired routine to stretch your entire body using slow, rhythmic, and mindful breathing, in and out through the nose, to promote relaxation.

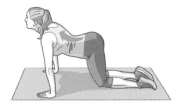

1.   Cat-Cow (5 breaths in and out) *page 70*

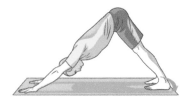

2.   Downward-Facing Dog (5 breaths in and out) *page 122*

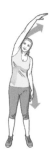

3.   Standing Crescent Moon (5 breaths in and out per side) *page 74*

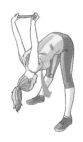

4.   Wide-Legged Forward Fold with Chest Expansion (5 breaths in and out) *page 108*

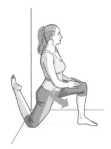

5.   Assisted Low Lunge (5 breaths in and out per side) *page 110*

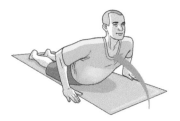

6.   Low Cobra (5 breaths in and out) *page 68*

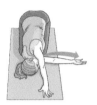

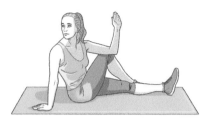

7. Thread the Needle (5 breaths in and out per side) *page 40*

8. Half Lord of the Fishes (5 breaths in and out per side) *page 88*

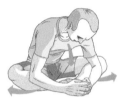

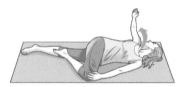

9. Bound Angle (5 breaths in and out) *page 90*

10. Supine Spinal Twist (5 breaths in and out per side) *page 72*

Rather than counting the number of seconds per stretch, focus on counting the cycles of breath (one cycle is a full inhalation and exhalation) to further emphasize the importance of proper breathing while stretching.

Roll and Stretch

In this routine, self-myofascial release is paired with static stretching to improve your tissue density and tissue length, which gets your entire body moving more efficiently. You'll use a foam roller for some of these exercises.

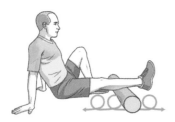

1. **Self-Myofascial Release for Calves** (60 seconds per side) *page 120*

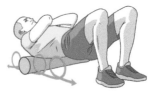

2. **Self-Myofascial Release for Mid and Upper Back** (60 seconds) *page 66*

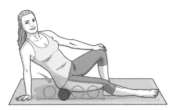

3. **Self-Myofascial Release for Glutes** (60 seconds per side) *page 94*

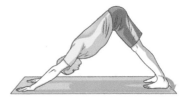

4. **Downward-Facing Dog** (60 seconds) *page 122*

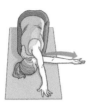

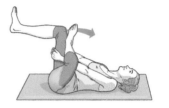

5. **Thread the Needle (60 seconds per side)**
page 40

6. **Figure 4 (60 seconds per side)** *page 92*

If you are pressed for time, simply perform each of the static stretches (stretches 4 through 6) for 30 seconds each.

Props and Support

To make stretching comfortable and more accessible, for this series of stretches I recommend using various props for support, such as a strap, towel, and a wall.

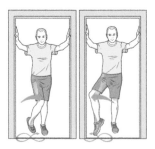

1. Figure 8 (8 repetitions per side) *page 98*

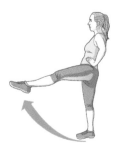

2. Leg Swings (10 repetitions per side) *page 96*

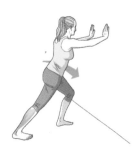

3. Standing Calf Stretch (30 seconds per side) *page 116*

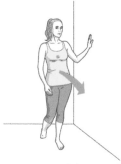

4. Tibialis Anterior Stretch (30 seconds per side) *page 118*

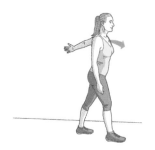

5. Biceps Stretch (30 seconds per side) *page 56*

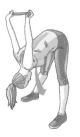

6. Wide-Legged Forward Fold with Chest Expansion (30 seconds) *page 108*

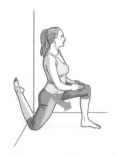

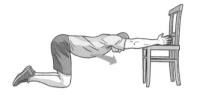

7. Assisted Low Lunge (30 seconds per side) *page 110*

8. Kneeling Lat Stretch (30 seconds) *page 78*

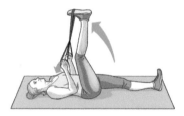

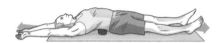

9. Assisted Supine Hamstring Stretch (30 seconds per side) *page 104*

10. Head-to-Toe Stretch (30 seconds) *page 80*

If you do not have a strap available for the Wide-Legged Forward Fold with Chest Expansion or the Assisted Supine Hamstring Stretch, use a small hand towel or belt as a substitute.

CHAPTER FOURTEEN

CUSTOMIZE YOUR WORKOUT

Be your own trainer! As you become familiar with the workouts in this book, challenge yourself to get creative and create your own workouts. You can start by following the workout structures I provide in chapters 10 through 13 and simply replace each move with one of the variations noted in the "Change It Up" section for each stretch. In addition to these variations, you can also develop your own stretching routine by mixing and matching the stretches from part 2 to meet your own needs and goals.

What Makes a Good Stretching Workout?

When creating your customized stretching workout, keep the following tips and principles in mind.

IDEALLY, HOLD STATIC STRETCHES FOR 60 SECONDS. Based on the current guidelines, you get the most benefit from each static stretch when you hold it for a total of 60 seconds. You can do this by breaking up the stretch, repeating it, say, 2 times for 30 seconds each or 4 times for 15 seconds each. If you want to vary your routine, one easy way to do that is to hold the stretches in the sequences for a total of 60 seconds each.

SEQUENCE YOUR DYNAMIC STRETCHES. When developing your workout of dynamic stretches, start with movements that go from front to back before moving to side-to-side movements and rotational movements.

CHOOSE A VARIATION THAT SERVES YOU BEST *TODAY*. Remember, your body is different every day, so when you're putting together a stretching routine, choose variations of the stretches that allow you to perform the movements without pain.

UNDERSTAND WHICH AREAS YOU ARE TRYING TO WORK. To make the most of your stretching workout, have a clear understanding of which areas of your body you are targeting with each stretch. Keep in mind that some stretches work multiple parts of your body, offering you more bang for your buck when designing your routine.

EXPLORE DIFFERENT STRETCHING TECHNIQUES. Although the routines in this book primarily focus on static and dynamic stretching, when creating your own workout, try other forms of stretching such as Active Isolated Stretching (AIS) and proprioceptive neuromuscular facilitation (PNF, see page 23), which both offer a host of benefits.

Working with a Professional

If you'd rather not go it alone on your stretching journey, enlist the professional guidance of a certified personal trainer who can create a customized stretching workout just for you, taking into account your unique fitness goals as well as other special considerations, such as any existing health conditions you might have. A knowledgeable personal trainer can also teach you the proper form for each stretch, making sure you get the most benefit from your workouts. Also, a personal trainer can provide a fun and motivational moving experience, helping to keep you accountable to a regular flexibility-training routine so you continue to make progress toward your goals.

Keep in mind, just like any profession, not all personal trainers are created equal. To find a professional who has earned a nationally accredited personal training certification, search the United States Registry of Exercise Professionals (USREPS): USreps.org.

RESOURCES

The following books, organizations, and their websites serve as trusted resources for providing further information on stretching and general health and fitness.

BOOKS

Biscontini, Lawrence. *The ABC's of Fitness: An Alphabet Guide to Wellness*. Delhi, India: FG2000, 2008.

Blahnik, Jay. *Full-Body Flexibility*. 2nd ed. Champaign, Illinois: Human Kinetics, 2010.

Freytag, Chris. *Move to Lose: Look and Feel Better in Just 10 Minutes a Day*. New York: Avery, 2004.

Martin, Cory. *Yoga for Beginners: Simple Yoga Poses to Calm Your Mind and Strengthen Your Body*. Berkeley, California: Althea Press, 2015.

Starrett, Kelly. *Deskbound: Standing Up to a Sitting World*. Las Vegas: Victory Belt, 2016.

ORGANIZATIONS AND THEIR WEBSITES

American College of Sports Medicine: ASCM.org

American Council on Exercise: AceFitness.org/acefit

National Academy of Sports Medicine: NASM.org

National Strength and Conditioning Association: NSCA.com

United States Registry of Exercise Professionals: USreps.org

REFERENCES

American College of Sports Medicine *ACSM's Guidelines for Exercise Testing and Prescription,* 9th ed. Philadelphia: Wolters Kluwer/Lippincott Williams & Wilkins, 2014.

Costa, Pablo B., Barbara S. Graves, Michael Whitehurst, and Patrick L. Jacobs. "The Acute Effects of Different Durations of Static Stretching on Dynamic Balance Performance." *Journal of Strength and Conditioning Research* 23, no. 1 (January 2009): 141–147. doi:10.1519/JSC.0b013e31818eb052.

González-Ravé, José M., Angela Sánchez-Gómez, and Daniel Juárez Santos-García. "Efficacy of Two Different Stretch Training Programs (Passive vs. Proprioceptive Neuromuscular Facilitation) on Shoulder and Hip Range of Motion in Older People." *Journal of Strength and Conditioning Research* 26, no. 4 (April 2012): 1045–1051. doi:10.1519/JSC.0b013e31822dd4dd.

Herman, Sonja L., and Derek T. Smith. "Four-Week Dynamic Stretching Warm-Up Intervention Elicits Longer-Term Performance Benefits." *Journal of Strength and Conditioning Research* 22, no. 4 (July 2008): 1286–1297. doi:10.1519/JSC.0b013e318173da50.

Khalil, T. M., S. S. Asfour, L. M. Martinez, S. M. Waly, R. S. Rosomoff, and H. L. Rosomoff. "Stretching in the Rehabilitation of Low-Back Pain Patients." *Spine 17,* no. 3 (March 1992): 311–317. www.ncbi.nlm .nih.gov/pubmed/1533060.

Misner, J. E., B. H. Massey, M. G. Bemben, S. Going, and J. Patrick. "Long-Term Effects of Exercise on the Range of Motion of Aging Women." *Journal of Orthopaedic & Sports Physical Therapy* 16, no. 1 (1992): 37–42. doi:10.2519/jospt.1992.16.1.37.

Park, S. H. "Effects of Passive Static Stretching on Blood Glucose Levels in Patients with Type 2 Diabetes Mellitus." *Journal of Physical Therapy Science* 27, no. 5 (May 2015): 1463–1465. doi:10.1589/ jpts.27.1463.

Ryan, E. D., T. J. Herda, P. B. Costa, J. M. Defreitas, T. W. Beck, J. Stout, and J. T. Cramer. "Determining the Minimum Number of Passive Stretches Necessary to Alter Musculotendinous Stiffness." *Journal of Sports Sciences* 27, no. 9 (July 2009): 957–961. doi:10.1080/02640410902998254.

Tekura, P., R. Nagarathnaa, S. Chametchaa, Alex Hankeya, and H. R. Nagendrab. "A Comprehensive Yoga Programs Improves Pain, Anxiety, and Depression in Chronic Low Back Pain Patients More than Exercise: An RCT. *Complementary Therapies in Medicine* 20, no. 3 (June 2012): 107–118. http:// dx.doi.org/10.1016/j.ctim.2011.12.009.

Weng, M. C., C. L. Lee, C. H. Chen, J. J. Hsu, W. D. Lee, M. H. Huang, and T. W. Chen. "Effects of Different Stretching Techniques on the Outcomes of Isokinetic Exercise in Patients with Knee Osteoarthritis." *Kaohsiung Journal of Medical Sciences* 25, no. 6 (June 2009): 306–15. doi:10.1016/S1607-551X(09)70521-2.

Ylinen, J., H. Kautiainen, K. Wirén, and A. Häkkinen. "Stretching Exercises vs. Manual Therapy in Treatment of Chronic Neck Pain: A Randomized, Controlled Cross-Over Trial." *Journal of Rehabilitation Medicine* 39, no. 2 (March 2007): 126–32. doi:10.2340/16501977-0015.

STRETCHES

WORKOUTS

INDEX